CANCER DIAGNOSIS IN PRIMARY CARE

For Elsevier:

Commissioning Editor: Alison Taylor
Development Editor: Catherine Jackson
Project Manager: Elouise Ball
Senior Designer: George Ajayi
Illustration Buyer: Merlyn Harvey
Illustrator: Antbits

CANCER DIAGNOSIS IN PRIMARY CARE

Edited by

William Hamilton BSc MD FRCP FRCGP

General Practitioner and Senior Research Fellow, Academic Unit of Primary Health Care, University of Bristol, Bristol

Tim J. Peters BSc MSc PhD CStat ILTM FFPH HonFRCSLT

Professor of Primary Care Health Services Research, Academic Unit of Primary Health Care, University of Bristol, Bristol

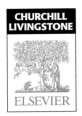

CHURCHILL LIVINGSTONE

ELSEVIER

EDINBURGH   LONDON   NEW YORK   OXFORD
PHILADELPHIA   ST LOUIS   SYDNEY   TORONTO   2007

CHURCHILL
LIVINGSTONE
ELSEVIER

© 2007, Elsevier Limited. All rights reserved.

First published 2007

No part of this publication may be reproduced, stored in a retrieval system, or transmitted in any form or by any means, electronic, mechanical, photocopying, recording or otherwise, without the prior permission of the Publishers. Permissions may be sought directly from Elsevier's Health Sciences Rights Department, 1600 John F. Kennedy Boulevard, Suite 1800, Philadelphia, PA 19103-2899, USA: phone: (+1) 215 239 3804; fax: (+1) 215 239 3805; or e-mail: healthpermissions@elsevier.com. You may also complete your request online via the Elsevier homepage (www.elsevier.com), by selecting 'Support and Contact' and then 'Copyright and Permission'.

ISBN-13: 978 0443 103674
ISBN-10: 0 443 10367 4

British Library Cataloguing in Publication Data
A catalogue record for this book is available from the British Library.

Library of Congress Cataloging in Publication Data
A catalog record for this book is available from the Library of Congress.

Note
Knowledge and best practice in this field are constantly changing. As new research and experience broaden our knowledge, changes in practice, treatment and drug therapy may become necessary or appropriate. Readers are advised to check the most current information provided (i) on procedures featured or (ii) by the manufacturer of each product to be administered, to verify the recommended dose or formula, the method and duration of administration, and contraindications. It is the responsibility of the practitioner, relying on their own experience and knowledge of the patient, to make diagnoses, to determine dosages and the best treatment for each individual patient, and to take all appropriate safety precautions. To the fullest extent of the law, neither the Publisher nor the Editors assume any liability for any injury and/or damage to persons or property arising out of or related to any use of the material contained in this book.

The Publisher

Working together to grow
libraries in developing countries

www.elsevier.com | www.bookaid.org | www.sabre.org

ELSEVIER   BOOK AID International   Sabre Foundation

ELSEVIER   your source for books, journals and multimedia in the health sciences
www.elsevierhealth.com

The publisher's policy is to use paper manufactured from sustainable forests

Printed in China

Contents

Contributors

Clare R. Bankhead BSc(Hons) MSc DPhil
Research Fellow, Department of Primary Care, University of Oxford, Oxford

Christine Campbell PhD MPH BSc(Hons)
Senior Research Fellow, General Practice, University of Edinburgh, Edinburgh

Roy Farquharson MD FRCOG
Clinical Director, Liverpool Women's Hospital, Liverpool

William Hamilton BSc MD FRCP FRCGP
General Practitioner and Senior Research Fellow, Academic Unit of Primary Health Care, University of Bristol, Bristol

Pippa Harris MBBS MRCP MRCGP
General Practitioner, Gateshead

Kirsten Hopkins MD MRCP FRCR
Consultant Oncologist, Bristol Oncology Centre, Bristol

David Kernick BSc MD FRCGP DA DCH DRCOG
General Practitioner, Exeter

Una Macleod MB ChB PhD MRCGP
General Practitioner and Senior Lecturer in General Practice, University of Glasgow, Glasgow

Elizabeth Mitchell BA PhD
Senior Lecturer in Research Methods, Glasgow Caledonian University, Glasgow

Richard D. Neal MB ChB MRCGP PhD
Clinical Senior Lecturer in General Practice, Cardiff University, Wrexham; General Practitioner, North Wales

Tim J. Peters BSc MSc PhD CStat ILTM FFPH HonFRCSLT
Professor of Primary Care Health Services Research, Academic Unit of Primary Health Care, University of Bristol, Bristol

Alison Round BSc FFPH MRCP
General Practitioner, Tiverton, Devon

Debbie Sharp MA BM BCh PhD FRCGP
General Practitioner and Professor, Academic Unit of Primary Health Care, University of Bristol, Bristol

Keith Sibson MB ChB MRCP
Specialist Registrar, Paediatric Oncology, Bristol Children's Hospital, Bristol

Jonathan Wallis FRCP FRCPath
Consultant Haematologist, Department of Haematology, Freeman Hospital, Newcastle-upon-Tyne

David Weller MB BS PhD FRACGP FRCGP MPH FAFPHM
General Practitioner and Professor of General Practice, Edinburgh

Clare Wilkinson MD MRCGP DRCOG
General Practitioner and Professor of Primary Health Care, School of Medicine, Cardiff University, Wrexham

Preface

A quarter of us will die of cancer, and most of these cancers are initially presented to primary care. Yet there is a remarkable shortage of information about how particular cancers present. Much of the information describes the symptoms of individual cancers. However, that is not how primary care works: patients consult with symptoms, not with cancers.

Therefore, the first decision was to try and turn the clinical problem around to start with a symptom. It has not always been possible, as almost any symptom can be cancer. The second decision was which cancers to include. We have chosen any cancer that a GP could expect to see once or more frequently in their clinical lifetime. The final decision was to make the book readable as well as factual. The editors' natural style is to write a 'fireside chat', yet the chapter authors (correctly) used a more scientific style. The first drafts of each chapter were heavily referenced, but we have reduced this to a short list at the end of each chapter. Although the 'fireside chat' style may have won, the facts should still be correct. We hope you enjoy it, as well as learning from it.

Willie Hamilton and Tim Peters

Acknowledgements

Our families and friends deserve particular thanks for listening to incessant stories of cancer diagnosis, and not telling us to get a life. Ian Daniels provided the clinical photographs – we wish you a most successful surgical career. Thanks are also due to the Medical Protection Society for the list of cancer-related cases they had managed, and to Cancer Research UK for the use of their statistics.

Chapter 1

Introduction
William Hamilton

The Importance of Cancer

Cancer is both an important and an emotional subject. It is important because approximately a quarter of people in the developed world die from it. Others suffer from cancer but are treated and survive. However, they are rarely able to be declared 'cured' as metastases can appear many years after the initial tumour has been treated. So, even if cancer is not a death sentence, it can be a life sentence of anxiety.

The emotional aspect of cancer relates to more than just its effect on mortality. People fear cancer. They fear cancer much more than they fear ischaemic heart disease, even though in many countries the latter causes more deaths. Furthermore, the prognoses of the two conditions are similar: rates of 5-year survival from angina and from breast cancer are very little different. Yet, if patients could somehow be given a choice between the two, few would opt for the cancer.

The Importance of Early Diagnosis of Cancer

It is generally believed that early diagnosis of cancer is beneficial. Of course, that's the reason why this book was written. This belief is widely and strongly held, probably because it seems so 'obvious' that diagnosing a cancer early is better than diagnosing it late. Most patients and their doctors consider that the gain to be had from early diagnosis is in terms of saving lives that would otherwise be lost. However, this is not the only possible benefit. Early diagnosis could be helpful in one of three main ways – or any combination of them. There may be a mortality benefit, a morbidity benefit or a psychological benefit.

Mortality

A cancer detected and treated at an early stage may be cured, whereas if it is identified only after it has metastasised the patient may (and usually will) die. Indeed, this reasoning is so self-evident that few studies have actually addressed whether early diagnosis is indeed helpful. There is another good reason for the lack of research into this aspect. The only way of testing if early diagnosis truly does provide a mortality benefit would be to design a randomised controlled trial incorporating a deliberate delay in one arm of the trial. This would raise major ethical problems, to say the least. There is, however, quite a lot of indirect evidence in favour of early diagnosis from screening or staging studies. Few would argue against the success of cervical screening, and the evidence is increasingly compelling for a mortality gain from mammography in breast cancer and faecal occult blood testing in colorectal cancer.

Staging studies also provide support for a mortality benefit from early diagnosis. Invariably, advanced stage cancers have a worse prognosis.* However, the relationship between the duration of symptoms and the stage of the cancer is complicated. In some cancers – breast and endometrial, for example – shorter durations of symptoms are associated with worse staging. There is no association between the duration of symptoms and the staging in cervical cancer. It may be that biologically aggressive tumours have only a short period of symptoms but are advanced at diagnosis.

The dearth of good research support for a mortality benefit from early cancer diagnosis has to be seen in context. It is impossible to assemble a case for delayed diagnosis. Even so, it is worth remembering that the public perception that early diagnosis of cancer *must* save lives is far ahead of the evidence.

Morbidity

A morbidity benefit from early diagnosis may arise in two main ways: earlier amelioration of symptoms or less extensive and/or invasive treatment. Given that most cancers are diagnosed at a symptomatic stage, and that treatment reduces or even eliminates symptoms, then earlier diagnosis

---

* A digression. An alternative term sometimes used for advanced stage cancer is late-stage cancer. It is late in one way – on the pathway from mutation of a single cell to the end result of a tumour metastasis, advanced-stage tumours are late. However, a synonym for 'late' is 'delayed'. Therefore, whether intended or not, describing a tumour as late stage implies that it could somehow have been identified earlier.

has obvious benefits. Furthermore, for several cancers the decision whether to augment surgery by radiotherapy or chemotherapy is influenced by the stage of the cancer. Given that both radiotherapy and chemotherapy can have undesirable side-effects, being able to have surgery alone may be a real benefit. Indeed, it is quite possible that the morbidity benefits from early diagnosis of symptomatic cancer outweigh the mortality benefits, even though, once again, they have not been proved.

Psychological Benefits

This comes back to the fact that patients fear cancer. Once the diagnosis has been raised as a possibility, patients wish to know if their fears are true or not. Even if the diagnosis does turn out to be malignant, patients value the resolution of their uncertainty. This is probably the principal gain to be had from the establishment of facilities offering rapid investigation of suspected cancer. In the UK the main forum for such investigation are the '2-week clinics'. These offer a facility whereby a patient whose GP** considers cancer as a possible cause of their symptoms can be seen by a specialist within a fortnight. Few people would argue that reducing the investigation time to 2 weeks is biologically essential; equally few would dispute the psychological benefits for speedy confirmation (or, more commonly, refutation) of the patient's fears.

Disadvantages of Cancer Diagnosis

All the above seems clear enough: diagnosing cancer is a good thing. However, it is possible to diagnose cancer, give treatment and yet not change the patient's long-term outlook. The most obvious example of this is prostate cancer. Screening for prostate cancer identifies some cancers that would never have become clinically apparent in the patient's lifetime. Currently, there is no reliable method of knowing which early prostate cancer will pose problems and which will not. Some of these men will have surgery with no mortality gain but a morbidity loss from treatment side-effects, let alone any psychological issues.

** We will use the abbreviation GP (general practitioner) throughout this book to mean the particular clinician managing the patient. This is not to disregard the possibility of other primary care clinicians being involved in the diagnosis of cancer: it can and does happen. However, the collective term 'primary health-care professional' is cumbersome and so we have chosen to avoid it.

Presentation of Cancer

Most cancers present initially to primary care, and most have symptoms. Alternative pathways exist, such as cancers detected by screening or emergency presentations. Some are never detected during the patient's lifetime, being found at post-mortem. The GP may have some input into these alternative pathways, such as cervical screening.

The mere fact that screening services exist alters the way in which some cancers present to primary care. It is not uncommon for the GP's first input to be when the patient comes to them with an abnormal result from screening, as with an abnormal prostate specific antigen (PSA) level taken at a company medical. In this case, the GP's role is largely just to refer the patient to the correct specialist. This doesn't require massive intellectual input from the GP, other than to design a watertight system for ensuring screening results are acted upon. However, the effect of screening services is to change the way cancers present. For instance, during a pilot study of colorectal cancer screening, the proportion of patients presenting with a surgical emergency fell in those accepting screening.

Therefore, screening is very relevant to primary care diagnosis of cancer and is covered in an early chapter in this book. Nonetheless, the commonest mode of cancer diagnosis for almost all cancers remains presentation to primary care with symptoms.

The Components of Primary Care Cancer Diagnosis

There are four steps in cancer diagnosis, shown schematically in Figure 1.1.

Considering Cancer as a Possibility

The first step is to consider cancer as a possibility at all. This may be easy – the patient may have presented with a lump in her breast. Whether or not she actually voices her fears that the lump may be malignant, the GP is very likely to consider cancer in the differential diagnosis.

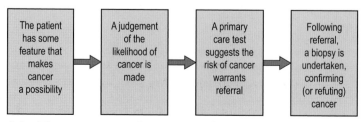

Figure 1.1   The components of primary care cancer diagnosis.

At the other end of the spectrum, many symptoms are not so clearly linked with cancer. Constipation is one example. If GPs were given a multiple-choice question 'Can colorectal cancer present with constipation?', all would answer 'yes'. The difficulty is when the question is turned around: 'What is the cause of my patient's constipation?'. If asked to list the possible diagnoses for constipation, a GP would probably include colorectal cancer in the top five, maybe after dietary change, drugs and medical conditions, such as hypothyroidism. The GP also knows that the other conditions are much more common; indeed, the most frequent outcome in primary care will be that no diagnosis will be made at all. Moreover, as benign conditions underlie the vast majority of complaints of constipation, primary care management of constipation concentrates on these. To some extent, the GP's experience of constipation being largely benign will *diminish* the prospect of identifying a cancer.

Over their clinical careers, GPs establish their own modus operandi for dealing with these common complaints. If this does not include investigating for cancer then, in practical terms, cancer has dropped off the GP's list of differential diagnoses for these common symptoms. In simple terms, if the GP doesn't think of cancer, then they won't diagnose cancer. So, one of the functions of this book is to describe the ways in which cancer can present.

Initial Judgement of Risk

Once the possibility, however remote, of cancer has been raised, the GP seeks to quantify the risk. This is generally by further history taking and examination, plus simple investigations. In most cases, the GP can fairly confidently rule out cancer. Indeed, the giving of appropriate reassurance is one of the core functions of general practice. Equally, it is one of the core functions of this book, so much so that it could alternatively have been titled 'How to *not* diagnose cancer in primary care'. So, a second function of this book is to describe (wherever possible) the risk of cancer with common symptoms. Diagnosis of cancer in primary care could be viewed as risk management. Should a GP mention the tiny possibility of cancer in a patient whose only complaint is fatigue? Should they investigate a patient whose cough has lasted 3 weeks? Risk management is a little easier when the size of the risk is known.

Primary Care Investigation for Cancer

In many cancers, once the possibility of a malignancy has been considered, a test can be ordered by the GP to refine the risk further. In the earlier question about a patient with persistent cough, the GP may order a chest X-ray. If this shows a pulmonary mass, the risk of cancer is now high enough to make specialist referral necessary. Alternatively, the X-ray may yield an intermediate result such as vague shadowing. Even in these cases, the investigative plan is usually straightforward (in this example it requires a repeat X-ray a few weeks later). Finally, the chest X-ray may be entirely normal, so the GP can reassure the patient (putting aside for a minute the risk of either a false negative from radiologist error or a tumour hidden by other intrathoracic structures). Similarly, in a man with urinary symptoms and a large prostate, a PSA test will help to decide if the enlargement is malignant.

In some cancers this middle stage is missing; for example, there is no intermediate stage in primary care diagnosis of breast cancer. However, once examination has revealed a lump then the risk of cancer is usually high enough to justify referral to a breast surgeon. With other cancers, a mass may also be palpable, as with some testicular, ovarian or head and neck cancers. It does not have to be a mass to raise the level of risk high enough to warrant referral: papilloedema in a patient with headache would certainly do so.

Of the common cancers, colorectal cancer is the trickiest in this respect. Some rectal cancers can be detected by rectal examination, some patients have iron deficiency anaemia, and a few have a positive faecal occult blood. The majority have 'softer' symptoms such as rectal bleeding, diarrhoea or abdominal pain, which individually carry a fairly low risk of cancer. Thus, many patients selected for investigation of possible colorectal cancer are actually at quite low risk of having cancer. This is in contrast to patients with a breast lump, pulmonary mass or a raised PSA, all of whom have at least a moderate chance of cancer. The overall yield of cancers in the referred population is therefore lowest for colorectal cancer; for the other cancers, the GP has effectively (and correctly) ruled out malignancy in many of the non-referred patients.

Definitive Diagnosis

The GP rarely makes the actual diagnosis of cancer. To do so requires a biopsy, which is not usually performed in primary care. The exception is excision biopsy of skin lesions, although few GPs would deliberately do an excision of a skin lesion if they suspected the skin lesion could be malignant.

GPs will often be able to make a confident clinical diagnosis of cancer. Many palpable tumours have a characteristic hardness, which makes an alternative diagnosis unlikely. Equally, a chest X-ray can be clearly malignant, and few enormously raised PSA results turn out to be from a benign prostate. Disseminated cancer can also give an unforgettable picture of cachexia. Nonetheless, as cancer is so important, histological diagnosis is almost always sought and this requires specialist referral. This book aims to help in deciding which patients require such referral.

Guidelines and the Selection of Patients for Referral

In the UK, other advice about selection of patients exists, notably the UK Referral Guidelines for Suspected Cancer. These were first published in 2000 covering England and Wales, with a Scottish version published 2 years later. They were updated in 2005. These documents describe particular symptoms or clinical presentations associated with cancer. For instance, the guidelines recommend urgent referral to a 2-week clinic in five possible presentations for lung cancer, seven for colorectal cancer and two for prostate cancer.

Undoubtedly, these guidelines are based on thorough, systematic reviews of the cancer literature.[+] However, very little of the research base originated in primary care and many of the recommendations have had to be derived from secondary care case series. Furthermore, even though the process of reviewing the literature was of the highest quality, it was necessary for the developers of the guidelines to make simple recommendations. A highly complex piece of guidance is much less likely to be used. However, this simplification of guidance leads to the concern that such guidelines are best at identifying the common presentations of cancer (which GPs believe they could spot anyway). As a result, common presentations of cancer are eased onto the investigation pathway of the 2-week clinic. This is a good thing but the countereffect is that patients with atypical presentations may be disadvantaged by being excluded from the same accelerated diagnostic pathway. Worse still, there are theoretical concerns that atypical cancers may be those with most to benefit from early diagnosis. For instance, a slow-growing colorectal cancer could simply give abdominal pain and constipation, and so fall outside the current guidance. Yet if this slow-growing cancer were to be identified early, spread may be prevented. Diagnosis of an obvious cancer with spread to the liver is undoubtedly important but has less mortality gain to offer.

[+] Indeed, the full version of the guidelines has a vast reference list at the end. We have taken the opposite view. We want this book to be read and we know the deadly effect that a list of references can have on readability.

A Threshold Risk for Referral

Neither this book nor guidelines can tell the GP whether a patient actually has cancer. Rather, guidelines are designed to assist them in identifying patients in whom the risk of cancer is high enough to warrant urgent investigation. This implies that there is a threshold level of risk mandating urgent investigation (and below which urgent investigation is not required). However, this threshold level is not made explicit in any of the guidelines. No doubt there were good reasons for this. One main reason for omitting to set a threshold level of risk for investigation is that patients have very different views about what level of risk they would choose. Some patients would decline investigation by colonoscopy if told they had a 2% risk of colorectal cancer (particularly once told of the small risk of perforation). Others would wish investigation however tiny the risk.

Furthermore, there is the issue of resources: chest X-rays and ultrasound scans are relatively cheap. Therefore, if the cancer can be identified by one of those, the threshold for ordering a test can be quite low. Conversely, colonoscopies consume quite a lot of resources (and cause the patient some discomfort) so there is an argument for having a higher threshold for requesting one.

To help our UK readers, we have given an abbreviated version of the UK guidelines early in each chapter. Where possible, we have given estimates of risk attributable to particular symptoms. This was only possible for a few cancers. Inevitably, our approach means that for some scenarios this book suggests referral, yet the UK guidelines do not – and vice versa. As always, the final decision is between doctor and patient. At least now it should be an informed one.

Chapter 2

Evaluating Risk – Concepts and Terminology

Tim J. Peters

Introduction

This chapter intends to define and explain briefly the epidemiological terms used in the remaining, more clinically oriented chapters. Although it is a stand-alone attempt at defining and explaining such terms, it is not designed as a comprehensive epidemiological/statistical reference for screening and diagnosis. Indeed, a reader well versed in the subject could skip the chapter entirely.

Consequently, this chapter will not provide definitions and explanations of terms such as likelihood ratios, Bayes' theorem, receiver operating characteristic curves and detailed aspects of clinical decision making such as utilities. Important as these concepts and methods are, for more thorough epidemiological coverage the interested reader is pointed in the direction of the many excellent general texts available. This chapter will, however, cover the following terms arranged under the broad issues to which they relate:

Prevalence and incidence will be defined as *measures of disease frequency*, followed by the *concept and evaluation of risk*. Next there are *measures of association* – in particular, risk ratios, odds ratios, risk differences and numbers needed to treat (NNTs) – and, briefly, the concepts of confounding and effect modification. Key *epidemiological study designs* such as cross-sectional, prospective cohort and retrospective case–control studies will then be described, together with randomised controlled trials (RCTs), including the concepts of efficacy, effectiveness and intention-to-treat analysis. *Performance statistics of diagnostic and screening tests* will be presented in detail – in particular the notions of false positives and false negatives, and measures of sensitivity, specificity, positive and negative predictive value (PPV and NPV), pretest and post-test probability. Broader concepts in screening will then be covered, in particular interval cancers and lead-time bias.

Measures of Disease Frequency

The two classic measures of disease frequency are prevalence and incidence, which should not be confused with one another, let alone used interchangeably. In brief, prevalence reflects the total amount of, quite literally, prevalent disease among a group of individuals at a given time, whereas incidence represents the occurrence of new observations of disease over a period of time in a given group of individuals.

Prevalence is therefore simply defined as the proportion of individuals with the condition and is expressed as a proportion, percentage or number per convenient radix (e.g. per 100,000) of individuals. For example, the prevalence of colorectal cancer in a UK general practice could be of the order of 0.05% or, equivalently, five cases per 10,000 list size. The prevalence of any disease, including cancer, will increase through a combination of large numbers of new cases and survivors of the condition.

Incidence, on the other hand, is defined as the number of new cases in a specified period of time (usually a year) divided by the number of individuals who could develop the condition in this period (multiplied again by a convenient radix such as 1000, 10,000 or 100,000). You can therefore spot a proper incidence if a figure is presented as, say, 'the incidence of breast cancer in women in the UK is 140 per 100,000 per year' or equivalently, that the annual incidence is 140 per 100,000. More commonly, you'll see disease frequencies quoted as 'incidence' rates either with (a) no time period stated or (b) no feasible time period involved. If so, then it is always worth ensuring that the terminology is correct, which it often won't be.

In general, prevalence is influenced by both the incidence and the duration of disease, with the duration determined by a combination of the cure and case-fatality rates. An analogy often drawn at this point is with a pool of water, with incidence reflected in the rate of flow into the pool and prevalence by the amount of water within it, which is itself determined by the flow into it and the flow out. Cancers which are comparatively readily and rapidly fatal (such as lung cancer) or commonly cured (basal cell carcinoma) will have a low prevalence over wide ranges of incidence. Conversely, slow developing and/or comparatively rarely fatal cancers with an equivocal 'cure' rate (such as prostate cancer) will have a higher prevalence than might be expected from their incidence.

The above definitions cover the measures as descriptive statistics but in real life all such quantities are usually calculated for samples rather than whole populations. As the figures arise from a sample, all such measures could (and usually should) be accompanied by confidence intervals. We have decided to omit these as our quoted figures are largely for illustration and comparison, however much this goes against the statistical grain.

The Concept and Evaluation of Risk

The definition of incidence means that this measure is more properly termed an *incidence rate*. Closely linked to this is a measure known as *cumulative incidence*, which is the proportion of new cases of disease in a period of time. This time period is usually fixed but can be variable, as with a lifetime incidence. A synonym for cumulative incidence is the *risk* of disease. Amazingly, epidemiological terminology actually coincides with what would generally be understood by a word. It is portrayed in the following formula:

$$\text{Risk} = \frac{\text{number of individuals experiencing the outcome in the time period}}{\text{number of individuals without the condition at the start}}$$

Examples of risk given in this book are: 1% of women with high-grade cervical intraepithelial neoplasia (CIN3) develop invasive cervical cancer per year (Chapter 12); the 3% risk of prostate cancer among men aged over 40 years who present with lower urinary tract symptoms (Chapter 8); and (to show risks can be for desirable outcomes) the 5-year survival of around 70% of women diagnosed with early-stage ovarian cancer (Chapter 10). Regarding the latter figure, a crucial question relates to how this compares with the 5-year survival for women diagnosed with advanced ovarian cancer, leading us to the next section.

Measures of Association

These concern epidemiological relationships between variables. This includes associations between possible risk factors and the development of disease – for example, between various dietary measures and the risks of stomach or prostate cancer. Other possible contexts are associations between stage of disease at diagnosis and survival, and measuring the impact of interventions such as adjuvant chemotherapy for breast cancer, in terms of disease recurrence.

In the following detailed definitions, the terminology of *exposure* and *outcome* is adopted for measures of association; in the above examples the first mentioned variables (diet, stage and therapy) are exposures and the second (cancer, survival and recurrence) the outcomes. For simplicity, all these outcomes are *binary* in that they have just two possible categories: you develop cancer or you do not; you survive or die; you have a recurrence or you do not.

The first conventional measure of association is the *risk ratio* (RR) or relative risk. This is obtained from the following formula:

$$RR = \frac{\text{risk of outcome among those exposed}}{\text{risk of outcome among those not exposed}}$$

If the exposure/risk factor increases risk then the RR will be over 1, and if it decreases risk then the RR is below 1. A closely related measure of association is provided from a recasting of the risk from a probability to an *odds*. The odds are derived by considering that if an outcome has, for example, a one-in-three chance of occurring, then the odds of the outcome are one-to-two; hence a risk of 0.333 translates to odds of 0.5. An alternative measure of association is therefore the *odds ratio* given by:

$$OR = \frac{\text{odds of outcome among those exposed}}{\text{odds of outcome among those not exposed}}$$

The odds ratio has some advantages over the risk ratio, which explain why it is seen more frequently in the literature (and this book) than would seem warranted. First, the odds ratio is the measure produced by *logistic regression*. In this technique, measures of association are investigated to see if they survive attempts to find other ('third-party' or *confounding*) variables that explain an apparent association between an exposure and an outcome, or if the association between the exposure and the outcome is different at different levels of another variable (*effect modification* or *interaction*).

Second, the OR can be obtained from a variety of the study designs described in the following section – in particular, prospective cohort and retrospective case–control studies – whereas the RR is not directly calculable from the latter. The reason for this is that the OR is 'symmetrical' in the sense that you get the same answer whether you calculate the ratio of the odds of the outcome given exposure status (as you would in a cohort study) or the ratio of the odds of exposure given outcome status (as in a case–control study). If the disease is rare then the OR and RR are very similar and so for most case–control studies the RR can at least be estimated approximately. Sadly, there is no simple rule of thumb for 'how rare is rare', since it depends on the magnitude of the association as well as the prevalence of the disease. Whilst in general numerically different from one another, the RR and the OR do share the above broad interpretations for values above or below 1, which for both measures is the value representing no association between exposure and outcome.

This is of course all a bit less of a problem if you are familiar with odds in betting, where for example if an Ulsterman offers an Englishman odds of 5:1 for a Northern Ireland versus England football match, then the implicit 'agreement' is that Northern Ireland have a one-in-six chance of winning the game.*

More formally, odds and risks (or probabilities) are related as follows:

$$\text{Odds} = \frac{\text{risk of outcome occurring}}{\text{risk of outcome not occurring}} \quad \text{or} \quad \frac{\text{risk of Northern Ireland winning (1 in 6)}}{\text{risk of England winning (5 in 6)}}$$

The two risks could simply be subtracted to obtain an absolute measure known, not surprisingly, as the *risk difference* (RD):

RD = risk of outcome among exposed – risk of outcome among unexposed

As well as having its own intuitive appeal, the RD can be used to derive the *number needed to treat* (NNT) to obtain one favourable outcome. For example, consider professional cricketers whose job demands long hours of sun exposure, and that sun-cream halves the lifetime risk of malignant melanoma from 1.5% to 0.75%. The risk difference is 0.75%, or 7.5 per 1000 individuals, and the NNT is about 134 (1000/7.5). Assuming that the evidence for sun-cream is robust (including that there are no confounding factors interfering with the above risk estimates), this means that for every 134 cricketers targeted, we would expect to avoid one malignant melanoma.

Study Designs

The main study designs in primary care cancer epidemiology comprise three observational (cross-sectional, cohort and case–control) and one experimental (randomised controlled trial) designs.

Cross-sectional studies are where exposures and outcomes are ascertained at the same point in time – for instance, from some combination of self-administered questionnaires and clinical or record examination. This design has advantages of speed and comparatively low cost but the disadvantage that the temporal order of the exposure and outcome is generally

---

* And they did – thanks for asking. This illustration ignores the remote possibility of a draw, which was rightly seen by both parties as impossible.

impossible to gauge. Both *prospective cohort studies* and *retrospective case–control studies* attempt to study individuals through time: the first forward in time, observing exposures as they occur and then awaiting outcomes later, sometimes much later; the second starting from those known to have the disease (the cases) or not (the controls) and ascertaining exposure retrospectively, assuming it is available and reliable. They therefore have advantages but also some disadvantages as apparent in their above descriptions.

Only in an experimental design such as the *randomised controlled trial* (RCT) can confounding be ultimately eliminated with any confidence, since random allocation to one intervention or another removes such biases. The RCT is generally held to be the 'gold standard' design for investigating *efficacy*, which is the effect of an intervention under ideal circumstances, as compared to *effectiveness*, which is its effect/impact in general use. Pragmatic RCTs involving comparatively liberal entry criteria and flexible 'real-life' protocols for the interventions are designed to obtain estimates of efficacy that most closely reflect effectiveness. This also requires RCTs to be (correctly) analysed on an *intention-to-treat* basis, where the groups as randomised are compared regardless of the extent of compliance with the intended interventions.

Performance Statistics

The above measures are all designed to represent the relationship between exposure and outcome for general epidemiological purposes. For screening and diagnosis, the predictive value of an exposure for the outcome of interest is what is wanted, with its 'performance statistics'. The exposure may be a test result but equally it could be the reporting of a symptom or a clinical examination finding. We want to know what a test result *really* means (does a 'negative' colonoscopy rule out colorectal cancer?) or what a symptom really means (does haemoptysis mean your patient has lung cancer?) or what an examination finding implies (are testicular masses cancerous?).

Sensitivity and Specificity

The main measures used when describing test results are the *sensitivity* and *specificity* of the (binary) test in relation to the (binary) outcome. The standard arrangement is depicted in Table 2.1, with sensitivity defined as the proportion of individuals with the disease who are (correctly) positive on the test, and specificity as the proportion of individuals who do not have the disease who are (correctly) negative on the test.

Table 2.1 Sensitivity, specificity, prevalence, positive predictive value (PPV) and negative predictive value (NPV)

Test/symptom	True disease state	
	Present	*Absent*
Positive	a	b
Negative	c	d

$$\text{sensitivity} = a/(a+c)$$

$$\text{specificity} = d/(b+d)$$

$$\text{prevalence} = (a+c)/(a+b+c+d)$$

$$\text{positive predictive value (PPV)} = a/(a+b)$$

$$\text{negative predictive value (NPV)} = d/(c+d)$$

High sensitivity means that most of those with the condition will be detected by the test and, commensurately, that there will be comparatively few individuals with the disease who are 'missed' by the test – that is, few *false negatives*. Clearly, a test that is literally 'sensitive' to the condition of interest is desirable if there is a high penalty in respect of health outcome for such missed diagnoses, including the issue of 'false reassurance' that might result in delay in reporting symptoms, delayed investigation/diagnosis, or both. High specificity reflects good ability to *exclude* the condition of interest (literally, how specific it is) and, commensurately, that there will be comparatively few individuals without the disease who are wrongly identified by the test as being 'at risk' – that is, few *false positives*. False positives in a screening programme are particularly unhelpful in that they lead to healthy (and usually asymptomatic) individuals being subjected to what can be expensive, lengthy and potentially risky procedures plus any concomitant anxiety.

Unfortunately, achieving a high sensitivity and high specificity simultaneously is difficult (indeed, all other things being equal, they will be inversely related) and even in the context of diagnosis it is unusual for the trade-off between the disadvantages of false positives and negatives to be straightforward. An analogy with a fishing net might help here: if its mesh is too wide then the targeted fish are more likely to be missed (increased risk of false negatives and reduced sensitivity); if it is too narrow then fish of a smaller size than required will be literally caught in the net (increased risk of false positives and reduced specificity).

Sensitivity and specificity are considered to be the fundamental measures of a test's performance and could be expected to be relatively constant in different circumstances.** This is not entirely true, since different laboratory procedures, equipment and staff, different patient populations and primary health-care circumstances will all lead to variations in test performance in practice. However, the prevalence of the disease should not alter the sensitivity or specificity (as they are calculated 'down the columns' of Table 2.1).

Predictive Values

The other two common performance statistics for diagnostic and screening tests are the *positive predictive value* (PPV) and the *negative predictive value* (NPV). These are defined formally in Table 2.1 but the PPV is the probability that an individual with a positive test result actually has the disease, and the NPV is the probability that an individual with a negative test result does not actually have the disease. While these are dependent on the prevalence – in particular, for a rare disease it is difficult to have a high PPV however good the test – they are the most helpful clinically for the GP and the patient. For example, against a background risk (prevalence) of 0.25%, presentation to the GP of a patient with rectal bleeding confers a PPV of 2.4%, a nearly 10-fold increase in risk for colorectal cancer.

The predictive values are therefore also crucial in deciding whether a specific test (or reporting of a symptom) will be useful in a particular population (with a given prevalence), since the PPV and (1-NPV) are the two *post-test probabilities* that can be compared directly with the prevalence itself, which is effectively the *pretest probability*. Similar profiles can be derived for combinations of symptoms, as shown, for example, in Chapters 6, 7 and 8.

Other Relevant Concepts

In screening but also in clinical practice, a correctly negative test at one time can be followed by development of cancer later. In screening, these are *interval cancers* – they make the ultimate assessment of a test's performance statistics a challenge. Another difficulty in considering the value of such tests is the concept known as *lead-time bias*. If, for example, women with early-stage ovarian cancer were to be detected by a screening programme, but without the earlier diagnosis leading to improved outcomes, the screening programme would appear to be beneficial as women whose cancer was

---

** To reinforce the distinction between these two measures, it may help to reflect that as a lover, Casanova was renowned for his sensitivity but clearly specificity was not his strong point.

detected by screening would have longer survival times after diagnosis. It reinforces two general messages related to screening in particular: first, that it is only worthwhile if amongst other criteria there is a treatment that is beneficial (especially if applied early); and second, RCTs with a comparison arm that does not receive screening are required to establish the ultimate effectiveness and cost-effectiveness of such programmes overall.

Further Reading/Key References

Fletcher R H, Fletcher S W, Wagner E H 1988 Clinical epidemiology. The essentials, 2nd edn. Williams and Wilkins, Baltimore

Kirkwood B R, Sterne J A C 2003 Essential medical statistics, 2nd edn. Blackwell Science, Oxford

Last J M 2001 A dictionary of epidemiology, 4th edn. Oxford University Press, Oxford

Peters T J, Wildschut H I J, Weiner C P 2006 Epidemiologic considerations in screening. In: Wildschut H I J, Weiner C P, Peters T J (eds) When to screen in obstetrics and gynecology, 2nd edn. Elsevier Saunders, Philadelphia

Chapter 3

Screening and Early Diagnosis of Cancer

Alison Round and David Weller

Introduction

All screening programmes do both harm and good, which contributes to the controversy that surrounds some of them. The aim of this chapter is not to review arguments for and against screening but to examine the significance of current, or proposed, cancer screening programmes in the UK for primary care, including the ways in which they may influence use of primary care services.

From an individual perspective, the point of screening is to reduce the risk of a particular disease or its complications. This is often equated with the performance of a particular test but clearly, screening is a programme, not just a test. All stages, and consequences, of the screening programme need to be taken into account. Ideally, the sensitivity and specificity should be quoted for the screening programme as an entirety, rather than for the screening test or tests alone. The programme's efficacy may vary considerably depending on factors such as uptake and screening intervals. Although the initial screening test, such as the measurement of prostate specific antigen (PSA), may be relatively unobtrusive and inexpensive, the investigations that follow a positive test are often invasive and anxiety provoking. Individuals who suffer adverse effects may have no prospect of benefit – if they do not actually have cancer or if they have a cancer that would not have troubled them during their lifetime. For breast, cervical and colorectal national cancer screening programmes, the judgement has been made that in the UK the overall benefits in terms of reduced mortality outweigh the harms engendered through the programme. Nevertheless, it is still true that those who benefit are not the same people as those who will suffer harm.

Table 3.1 Outcomes from screening

	Beneficial outcome	**Detrimental outcome**
Screening test positive	Early identification of disease, or risk of disease, which leads to early treatment and a better outcome	False identification of possible cancer, which can lead to anxiety, additional investigations, and even occasionally treatment Cancer identified that is not treatable or for which treatment has no impact on outcome Cancer identified that would have spontaneously regressed or not progressed further
Screening test negative	Reassurance that no cancer is present	False reassurance when cancer does exist but is not detected Reassurance that cancer is not present so no incentive to change individual behaviour (e.g. smoking cessation, dietary change) and reduce subsequent risk
Test offer not accepted		Anxiety raised by offer of test Feeling of regret and/or guilt if cancer subsequently diagnosed

For other cancers, the evidence that benefit outweighs harm is less convincing. So how does a GP advise on screening which is not part of a national programme (such as commercially available tests, often accessed via the internet)? Table 3.1 shows some of the possible 'good' and 'bad' outcomes. It may be helpful to talk these issues through with the patient before undertaking the test and, if possible, give some idea of the probabilities of the various outcomes, both beneficial and detrimental. This will be discussed further in the sections below on the individual cancers.

Breast Cancer

The UK mammography programme was established in 1988. Initially targeted every 3 years at women aged 50–65, it has now been extended to women up to the age of 70, and those over the age of 70 may still request mammography. Mammography is approximately 70–80% sensitive and 90% specific in postmenopausal women. The incidence of new cancers has increased since the screening programme started. This is partly due to increased diagnosis of ductal carcinoma in situ, which now accounts for 88% of all new breast cancers identified mammographically. Perhaps surprisingly, only 23% of all new cancers in the UK are diagnosed via the screening programme. The remainder are diagnosed on clinical grounds.

Survival has increased over the past 20 years, with 5-year survival being approximately 97% for those with localised disease, 77% for those with regional disease and 21% for those women with metastatic disease. The increase in survival is partly attributable to screening but undoubtedly, a large impact has been made by improved treatment with the routine use of adjuvant therapy, such as tamoxifen.

Other Potential Breast Screening Tests

Other types of breast screening have been proposed. Regular breast examination has not been demonstrated to reduce mortality in any study, and the sensitivity of detection is likely to be much lower in routine practice than

Table 3.2 Outcomes from mammography screening

	Beneficial outcome	**Detrimental outcome**
Mammography positive	23% of all cancers are diagnosed by this route – 7.9/1000 women screened 42% of these cancers are invasive yet small – 3.3/1000 women screened	51.4/1000 women undergo further assessment 18.3/1000 proceed to cytology or biopsy. The benign biopsy rate is 2.3/1000 women screened It is unknown how many cancers are already metastatic at diagnosis 21% of cancers diagnosed are not invasive or microinvasive –1.7/1000 women screened
Mammography negative	948.6/1000 women screened are reassured that no cancer exists	The number of interval cancers (i.e. those diagnosed in between screening rounds) varies; it is between 60% and 80% of the expected annual incidence rate by the third year of the programme
Test offer not accepted	Approximately 120/1000 women	12.8% women never have screening, and 24% refuse screening in any one screening round 1.9/1000 women may have a cancer that would be picked up if they were screened

in a trial. A Cochrane systematic review of breast self-examination concluded that no mortality benefit was seen despite the number of breast biopsies doubling. Magnetic resonance imaging (MRI) may have a higher sensitivity than mammography but a lower specificity, so will detect more cases of cancer at the cost of more false-positive test results. No randomised trials have been performed using MRI as a screening tool and the effect of repeated MRI examinations on the breast is not known. Likewise, there are no data for the use of ultrasound in a general population, and it probably also has a high false-positive rate.

Genetic testing is a further possibility; clinically significant BRCA mutations occur in 1:400 people and are associated with a greatly increased risk of breast and ovarian cancer. Requests for genetic testing are increasing. Screening for the BRCA1 and BRCA2 genes is a complex and costly process, requiring the assessment of risk of gene carriage, followed by genetic testing itself. The former is a clinical assessment of familial factors such as the age at breast cancer diagnosis, bilateral breast cancers, a history of both breast and ovarian cancer, multiple cases of breast cancer in a family and/or Ashkenazi Jewish heritage. Genetic testing is by DNA sequencing, with test results that can be negative, positive or uncertain (the latter in around 10% of cases). Once an abnormal gene has been detected, there is no consensus on what intervention should be offered. Even yearly mammograms may be insufficient to detect the highly proliferative cancer that occurs with BRCA mutations, and a programme of annual MRI, mammography and ultrasound scans together with twice-yearly clinical examination has been suggested.

Evaluation of the potential harms and benefits of a genetic screening programme for breast cancer has not been carried out. No mortality benefit has been demonstrated – in particular for chemoprevention with tamoxifen for women at high risk of breast cancer, since any reduction in the latter is balanced by adverse effects such as stroke and pulmonary embolism. There is no good evidence describing the adverse effects of bilateral prophylactic mastectomy, although breast cancer risk is considerably reduced.

Key Points

- General practitioners still diagnose the majority of breast cancers in the UK.
- Mammography remains the best evaluated and only screening modality to demonstrate mortality reductions.
- Regular breast self-examination cannot be recommended as an alternative to mammography.
- Screening for BRCA mutations cannot be recommended at present.

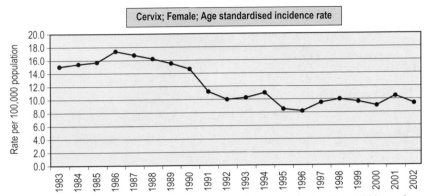

Figure 3.1 Annual incidence of new cervical cancers in the South West of England 1983–2002.
Data source: South West Cancer Intelligence Service.

Cervical Cancer

Cervical cancer develops slowly, with a long natural phase from preinvasive to invasive disease. Squamous carcinoma accounts for 90% of cervical cancers. It is strongly associated with human papilloma virus infection, which is sexually transmitted. The cervical cancer screening programme is unusual in that it detects precancerous lesions and hence prevents the development of actual cancer.

Despite a lack of randomised trial evidence, a national screening programme has been in place since 1988, consisting of 3- or 5-yearly cervical smears. Successful incentives to increase smear uptake were introduced in 1990, with a corresponding decrease in cancer incidence (Figure 3.1) and a decrease in mortality. However, a quarter of cervical cancers in the UK occur amongst those aged over 70 and so fall outside the screening programme. Liquid-based cytology is now the recommended detection method (although its superiority over conventional techniques remains contentious); even so, it still has a relatively poor sensitivity of 60–70% and a specificity of about 80%. Of all cervical smears, 3.3% have borderline changes, 1.6% mild changes and 1% moderate or severe changes.

Other Potential Screening Tests

Almost all cases of cervical cancer contain a type of human papilloma virus (HPV). Screening by HPV testing is more sensitive than cytology (80%) but less specific (78%), so a higher proportion of women will test positive and require colposcopy. This will be even higher in young women, who may have transient HPV infections but in whom the incidence of cervical cancer

Table 3.3   Outcomes from cervical screening

	Beneficial outcome	Detrimental outcome
Test positive	Unknown what percentage of all cancers are diagnosed by this route Less than 0.1% of all cervical screening tests identify a cancer 1% find moderate or severe cytological abnormalities ('changes') that may or may not be cancerous	9% of women undergo further assessment and 8% (~120,000 women per year) have colposcopy, of which only 2% (~2300 women per year) reveal cancer or precancer Of those with moderate or severe changes, 25% do not have cancer or precancer on further investigation Of those with repeated mild abnormality, 83% do not have cancer or precancer Some cancers diagnosed by cytology are not invasive or would have spontaneously regressed Some cancers are already metastatic at diagnosis
Test negative	91% of women screened are reassured that no cancer exists	The number of interval cancers varies with age. In women over 55, only 17% of cancers are interval, compared to ~39% of cancers in women under 40 1–2% of women have an inadequate result on their initial test with LBC
Test offer not accepted	19% of population offered screening do not accept, the majority of whom will not have cancer	Overall, 23% of all cancers in the appropriate age group are not diagnosed through the screening programme

is very low. HPV testing has been associated with heightened anxiety, even in those with a negative result. There is the potential for stigmatisation and partner discord. Large-scale studies are under way to consider the effectiveness of a papilloma virus vaccine.

Key Points

- The cervical screening programme and high levels of uptake appear to have decreased the incidence and mortality from cervical cancer.
- Almost 1 in 10 of women on the screening programme undergoes colposcopy. However, this may be less anxiety provoking than multiple repeated smears.

- HPV testing may be viable in the future, either as a basic screening test or as an adjunct to abnormal cytological findings.

Colorectal Cancer

The incidence of bowel cancer in the UK is amongst the highest in the world. Nevertheless, survival rates in the UK have improved over the past 25 years, and about half of people with newly diagnosed bowel cancer will still be alive in 5 years' time. Efforts to tackle this disease have focused on early diagnosis and screening, although recently there have also been significant improvements in treatment. There is good evidence supporting screening for bowel cancer, and it is likely to be an increasing feature in health care over the next several years. Guaiac-based testing of faecal occult blood is so far the only method of screening that has been shown to reduce disease-specific mortality; several trials have demonstrated reductions in colorectal cancer mortality of about 17% in groups of people who are offered screening using the faecal occult blood testing (FOBT).

A UK pilot of screening using FOBT was established in 2000; it demonstrated that a population-based programme could produce rates of uptake, test performance and pathology detected similar to those achieved in randomised controlled trials. The pilot has now completed two rounds of screening in England and Scotland.

Health ministers in both England and Scotland have committed to a national programme of screening for colorectal cancer, beginning in 2006. Screening will follow a similar pattern to that established in the pilot – that is, there will be a number of screening centres ('hubs') that will co-ordinate the programme, including invitations and follow-up, with endoscopy and other diagnostic and treatment services provided at more local and regional levels. At present there is considerable activity in increasing capacity for colonoscopy, pathology and other services associated with the provision of colorectal cancer screening. There is also a great deal of work being under-taken to establish adequate information technology and quality assurance systems.

There are several important challenges for primary care with the initiation of this programme; the pilot demonstrated that, while general practices are not directly involved in recruitment to screening, they do have important roles in co-ordination and information provision, leading to modest but real impacts on workload. Many people who take up an offer of screening are likely to be symptomatic. Bowel symptoms are highly prevalent in the UK population and there can be misconceptions about the use of screening tests such as the FOBT; they are not an alternative to seeking medical care for symptoms and, indeed, might provide false reassurance in such circumstances. Primary care has a role to play in educating patients about the strengths and limitations of this new programme; it will also have a key role in promoting uptake in hard-to-reach groups including those from socio-economically deprived backgrounds, males, those in younger age groups, and certain ethnic groups.

Table 3.4   Outcomes from colorectal screening

	Beneficial outcome	Detrimental outcome
Screening test positive	FOBT has a sensitivity of between 40% and 70% FOBT is not highly specific for cancer and it therefore has a low positive predictive value – only about 10% of positive results will lead to a diagnosis of cancer (this figure is higher if precancerous lesions such as adenomas are counted)	High false-positive rates, leading to many unnecessary colonoscopies Although rates of complication and death are extremely low from colonoscopy, particularly with current quality assurance measures, widespread screening will inevitably lead to accumulating adverse outcomes Screening also identifies much pathology which requires ongoing surveillance; while not necessarily a 'bad outcome', surveillance colonoscopies impose a very heavy workload on already stretched endoscopy services
Screening test negative	Reassurance that no cancer is present	FOBT misses about 40% of cancers; it is important that those screened remain diligent about responding to bowel symptoms despite a negative test
Test offer not accepted	In the pilot, uptake rates of about 58% were achieved, although this varied considerably according to various sociodemographic characteristics There is some evidence that uptake may drop off in subsequent rounds	A positive FOBT does induce anxiety, although this is generally shortlived

Other Potential Screening Tests

There is interest in refinements to the standard guiaic-based FOBT, particularly the immunochemical test. As yet, it is not known whether these newer tests would perform better in a national programme. There is also growing interest in the use of flexible sigmoidoscopy, particularly as this is a screening modality that could be delivered in primary care. A randomised study of flexible sigmoidoscopy screening will report in the near future.

Key Points

- The colorectal screening programme begins in 2006. Although separate from general practice, it is likely to generate some queries for GPs.
- Around one patient in 10 with a positive faecal occult blood will prove to have cancer.
- The benefits from screening may take some years to accrue, as removal of polyps may prevent cancers in future years.

Prostate Cancer

The natural history of prostate cancer is not well understood, and can vary greatly from aggressive invasive disease to very indolent tumours that do not contribute to morbidity and mortality. By the age of 80, 60–70% of men will have some cancer cells in their prostate, yet only 4% will die of prostate cancer. The number of deaths from prostate cancer in the UK has remained relatively stable over the past 15 years despite a doubling in incidence (Figures 3.2 and 3.3; data from South West Region, UK). In broad terms, a 50-year-old male has, over a lifetime, a 10% chance of being diagnosed with prostate cancer, with a 4% chance of death from it. The introduction of prostate cancer screening would increase the chance of a lifetime diagnosis to about 20%, but there is no good evidence that there would be any reduction in the risk of death. At present about 8% of cancers in the UK are diagnosed as a result of asymptomatic testing; in countries where PSA testing is much more widespread, about 30–75% of cancers are identified through this route.

The increase in incidence is largely due to the increase in prostate specific antigen (PSA) testing, which is being used in some places as a screening tool even though no screening programme is in place in the UK. Instead, there is a prostate cancer risk management programme, which indicates that PSA testing can be performed provided the man fully understands the lack of good-quality evidence for the risks and benefits of

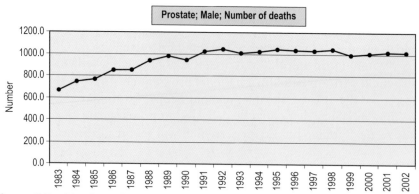

Figure 3.2   Number of deaths from prostate cancer in the South West of England 1983–2002.
Data source: South West Cancer Intelligence Service.

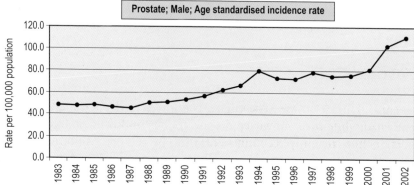

Figure 3.3   Annual incidence of prostate cancer in the South West of England 1983–2002.
Data source: South West Cancer Intelligence Service.

testing. Within this programme, there should be a standardised pathway for men whose test result is above the threshold.

The sensitivity of PSA (using a threshold level of 4 ng/ml) is about 70%, so an elevated PSA is not diagnostic of cancer. An ultrasound-guided prostate biopsy is required to establish the diagnosis. This may miss the tumour and is itself only about 80% sensitive. A large randomised study of prostate screening and treatment (the CAP and ProtecT trials) is under way in the UK.

Risk Factors/Future Advances

There is a genetic component to prostate cancer. The risk increases if relatives are diagnosed at an early age; with three affected relatives, the risk

Table 3.5   Outcomes from prostate screening

	Beneficial outcome	Detrimental outcome
PSA positive	Early cancer detected in 2.6% of men, and treatment may affect eventual outcome (there is some evidence for a small improvement in mortality with surgery for early prostate cancer though this remains uncertain)	10% of men undergo prostate biopsy (negative in 74% of cases); 10% of those with negative biopsies later turn out to have cancer It is unknown how many men have cancer detected that would not have otherwise affected them Treatment may lead to impotence (20–80%), incontinence (4–21%) or other impaired quality of life
PSA negative	90% of men reassured that no cancer present	0.7% of men who are tested have prostate cancer that is missed (20% of all prostate cancers) although in some cases this would not otherwise have affected them Anxiety and short-term stress experienced by up to 50% of men

is increased 7–10 times. African-American men have about twice the risk of those of white race. However, even with a strong genetic risk, active case finding is not currently recommended in the UK. There is no fundamental link with benign prostatic hyperplasia (BPH), although men with BPH often have a PSA taken, identifying a cancer.

Key Points

PSA testing is not currently recommended as a screening test, even in those with an increased genetic risk, because there is insufficient evidence that this will lead to improved survival from prostate cancer. Further research is under way.

Other Cancers for which Screening has been Proposed

Ovarian cancer

Ovarian cancer is relatively rare, with a low 5-year survival rate of between 30% and 50%. It typically presents quite late. Screening programmes have the potential to be worthwhile if it proves possible to detect the cancer at an early enough stage to apply effective treatment. However, no screening test has yet been identified that can reliably detect early-stage disease in the general population.

Two screening tests have been proposed: measurement of blood levels of CA-125, and transvaginal ultrasound. Both have only moderate sensitivities of 40–60%, reasonable specificities of 90–95%, and positive predictive values of about 20%. Even in high-risk women (those with genetic or hereditary risk factors), it is not clear whether the tests perform sufficiently well in detecting early-stage disease. Randomised controlled trials are under way.

Lung Cancer

Lung cancer has a high mortality, with survival being linked to stage at diagnosis. Five-year survival in stage 1 lung cancer is 70%, compared to overall figures of approximately 10%. Early diagnosis is the goal but no randomised trials have shown a mortality benefit from screening. Chest radiography and/or sputum cytology have been investigated in four randomised trials. The two that used radiography demonstrated both length- and lead-time bias, an apparent improvement in stage and survival from cancer, but with overall mortality unchanged between the screened and control groups. Spiral CT has been suggested as a screening test and 50,000 patients have enrolled in a large American study, due to report in 2009.

Bladder Cancer

Bladder cancer has an incidence of 20 new cases per 100,000 population per year. Approximately 80% of tumours are superficial and have a good prognosis, although they require regular follow-up. However, invasive tumours have a poor prognosis.

Several urine tests have been proposed as potential screening tests. Cohort studies of microscopic haematuria dipstick testing suggest that sensitivity and specificity are relatively poor: 20% of people have an initial positive test and would require cystoscopy, and of these, only 5% will have a cancer. The positive predictive value of microscopic haematuria for bladder cancer in the screened population is only 0.2% and this, combined with the relatively invasive diagnostic test of cystoscopy, makes a screening programme unattractive. Urine cytology has high specificity but poor sensitivity. The additional use of biological markers in the urine such as fibronectin can increase the sensitivity while maintaining a high specificity. Other studies have examined a molecule named MMP-9 but as yet, this has not progressed beyond very preliminary trials. However, there is no RCT evidence that using any of these techniques in an organised screening programme will improve mortality.

Further Reading/Key References

Atkin W S, Edwards R, Wardle J et al 2001 Design of a multicentre randomised trial to evaluate flexible sigmoidoscopy in colorectal cancer screening. Journal of Medical Screening 8(3):137–144

Jepson R, Weller D, Alexander F, Walker J 2005 Impact of UK colorectal cancer screening pilot on primary care. British Journal of General Practice 55:20–25

Towler B, Irwig L, Glasziou P et al 1998 A systematic review of the effects of screening for colorectal cancer using the faecal occult blood test, Hemoccult. British Medical Journal 317: 559–565

UK Colorectal Cancer Screening Pilot Group 2004 Results of the first round of a demonstration pilot of screening for colorectal cancer in the United Kingdom. British Medical Journal 329:133–138

Weller D, Alexander F, Orbell S et al 2003 Evaluation of the UK Colorectal Cancer Screening Pilot. A report for the UK Department of Health. Available online at: www.cancerscreening.nhs.uk/colorectal/finalreport.pdf

Chapter 4

Non-Specific Symptoms
William Hamilton and Debbie Sharp

Introduction

Most symptoms of cancer are specific to a single cancer, or at least give a clue as to which body system may be the source of the problem. Thus a symptom such as dysphagia immediately suggests an oesophageal problem, or postmenopausal bleeding a uterine problem. When faced with such a symptom, it is relatively easy for the GP to focus their diagnostic efforts on the suspected organ or organs.

Some other symptoms of cancer do not have an obvious link to one cancer site. In addition, these general symptoms of cancer, such as fatigue or weight loss, also frequently occur with benign conditions. So not only has the GP to consider if cancer is a possible diagnosis, he or she also has to think of where in the body the cancer may be, so that targeted initial investigation can take place.

Furthermore, some patients with cancer – especially lung cancer – just feel unwell. This feeling of general malaise is impossible to quantify (and difficult for patients to describe, or doctors to classify) but is nonetheless real. Many patients, after their diagnosis is made, are able to say, 'I knew there was something wrong'.*

It is not only primary cancers that can share common symptoms. For example, many cancers metastasise to bone and it is not uncommon for the initial presentation to be from the secondary spread to bone rather than from the primary tumour. In some instances, the secondary spread may mimic a primary cancer. A lung cancer secondary in the brain may present

---

* It is impossible to research the expression, 'I feel ghastly'. The only solution to this problem is for the doctor to listen to the patient. If they think there is something wrong, there usually is. Note that we say usually, not always.

very similarly to a primary brain tumour. Abnormal masses on a chest X-ray (CXR) may be primary or secondary cancers – indeed, they may be benign.

These non-specific presentations of cancer are dealt with in this chapter, along with simple investigations such as the erythrocyte sedimentation rate (ESR) and C-reactive protein (CRP) that may be used by GPs in this situation.

Weight Loss

Weight loss is a common symptom in patients with cancer. Around a quarter of patients with colorectal cancer or lung cancer report weight loss to their GPs at some time before diagnosis. It is much less common in prostate cancer or breast cancer, where it is really only reported by patients with advanced disease. The link between weight loss and cancer is complicated by the fact that some cancers (such as breast or colorectal) are more common in overweight patients. Indeed, the risk of breast cancer is lower in women who have deliberately lost weight during their adulthood.

The main issue is that it is *unintentional* weight loss that gives a clue to the possibility of an underlying cancer. Very few studies have defined what level of unintentional weight loss is enough to suggest cancer. Those that have set a threshold level have chosen different figures, usually in the range 5–10% of total body weight.

One problem is that loss of weight is fairly common in primary care. When 5200 unselected primary care attenders in Sweden were asked about possible cancer symptoms, 30 (0.6%) of them reported weight loss. However, it was not clear whether these 30 were actually proposing to discuss their weight loss at the consultation. A further problem in deciding whether – and how – to investigate weight loss is that the frequency of the various possible causes in primary care is unknown. In secondary care, about one-third of patients referred for investigation of *isolated* weight loss prove to have cancer. This figure comes from a large study of 328 patients. However, this was a highly selected group, in that they had been referred (so the GP was worried) and their weight loss was unexplained, there being no other clues to a diagnosis in the history, examination or primary care investigations. Even in that highly selected group, the only additional markers of a cancer diagnosis were being older, having a raised white cell count or abnormal liver function tests.

Isolated weight loss is a relatively rare primary care complaint, so this high chance of malignancy is unlikely to be typical of the average patient describing weight loss to their GP. Most such patients will have other symptoms that provide clues to the diagnosis, either malignant or benign, allowing the GP to narrow down the differential diagnoses. The exception to this is prostate cancer, when disseminated cancer may simply present as isolated weight loss.

> ### Box 4.1 Questions in a patient with unintentional loss of weight
>
> - How much weight has been lost?
> - Over what time period has the weight loss occurred?
> - What other symptoms are present?

The Risk of Cancer in a Patient with Weight Loss

When a patient aged between 40 and 70 years describes loss of weight to their GP, the approximate risk of cancer is between 1% and 2%. Colorectal cancer is the most common malignant cause, followed by lung cancer. Over the age of 70, the overall risk of cancer is much higher, around 10%, with colorectal, breast, lung and prostate cancers being approximately equally likely.

In patients who already have had a primary cancer, weight loss can be the sole symptom of recurrence. However, this should not be overinterpreted. In the physical and emotional aftermath of cancer diagnosis and treatment, weight loss is common even without a recurrence. In a study of women after treatment for early breast cancer, one woman in 10 who did *not* have a recurrence of their cancer had lost at least 6% of their body weight during the follow-up period. Nonetheless, weight loss was more common in those whose cancer had recurred.

How Much Weight has been Lost?

This is simply a guide to the seriousness of the symptom. It is reasonable to assume that the risk rises as the weight falls, and that a 10% loss of weight warrants fairly extensive investigation for possible cancer.

Over What Time Period has the Weight Loss Occurred?

Again this is only a rough guide. Malignant loss of weight, which is usually accompanied by loss of appetite, is a fairly rapidly progressive symptom. It usually (but not always) represents advanced-stage disease and once the cycle of weight loss and appetite loss is established, considerable amounts of weight can be lost in a short time. In contrast, slow loss of weight over several months is more likely to be due to a non-malignant cause.

What Other Symptoms are Present?

This is potentially a very long list. Loss of weight can be due to any cancer, especially one that has disseminated. It may be a particular feature in cancers of the gastrointestinal tract, particularly pancreatic cancer. Over half of patients with malignant loss of weight will have colorectal, lung, prostate or gastro-oesophageal cancer, so history taking will focus on these possibilities. Of course, as a non-malignant cause is more likely than a malignant one, questions also need to cover benign causes.

Assuming the history has given no clue to a possible cancer site, examination will look for clubbing, breast, abdominal or rectal masses, lymphadenopathy or an abnormal prostate. If there are still no clues from the history or examination, the GP will need to consider how best to investigate the loss of weight.

All these tests are simple and, together, should go a long way towards identifying the main malignant causes of weight loss. Furthermore, they should identify most benign causes. A finding of iron deficiency may be due to a caecal cancer; equally, it may be due to malabsorption, nutritional deficiency or several other causes. A raised blood sugar may explain the weight loss, though type II diabetes rarely presents as the classic triad of polyuria, thirst and weight loss. Abnormal liver or renal function tests may not exactly pinpoint the diagnosis. They will, however, guide management – such as suggesting an abdominal ultrasound or referral for specialist opinion. A prostate cancer severe enough to cause loss of weight will almost always have a (very) raised PSA. Similarly, a chest X-ray will usually reveal a lung cancer, though negative chest X-rays occur in a sixth or more of lung cancers. Finally, a positive faecal occult blood may be the only feature of a slowly growing colorectal cancer.

Fatigue

Fatigue is a very common complaint and encompasses a range of different concepts, from tiredness to the inability to perform one's usual activities. One in five adults report they have experienced tiredness in the previous 2 weeks, and around 2% of the adult population consult their GP with

---

Box 4.2   Investigation of weight loss without other features

- Full blood count, plus ESR or CRP
- Blood sugar
- Liver and renal function tests
- PSA
- Chest X-ray
- Faecal occult blood

fatigue in any one year. In older people, consultation for fatigue is even more common, with 3% of men and 7% of women over 75 years visiting their GP in any one year complaining of this symptom. With such high figures in the normal population it is not surprising that the risk of cancer is very low in patients complaining of fatigue. An elegant Dutch study recorded all malignancies diagnosed after a presentation of fatigue to primary care: in the 4 years after the symptom was reported to the GP, 3.7% of those with fatigue had developed a malignancy. This sounds high but reflected the age group studied; 3.4% of patients who had *not* complained of tiredness also developed a malignancy during the same 4 years.

Of the most common cancers, lung has the strongest association with fatigue. Over a third of patients report fatigue to their GP before diagnosis. Furthermore, a small proportion of lung cancer patients describe isolated fatigue for many months before diagnosis. Colorectal cancer may also present with fatigue, but in most instances it can be explained by the associated anaemia. Many haematological malignancies can cause fatigue; again, this is partly mediated through anaemia.

The Risk of Cancer in a Patient with Fatigue

The risk of cancer in a patient complaining of fatigue, and who has no other features of cancer, is very low. Overall, the risk is a little below 1% for patients under 70; however, most of the patients with cancer will have some other symptom providing a clue to the diagnosis. In patients over 70, the risk is approximately 2.5%. Many older patients complaining of fatigue will have anaemia as the initial explanation for their symptom, and this will need further investigation (see Chapter 6 on colorectal cancer).

How Long has the Fatigue been Present?

Again this is only a rough guide. It is probably sensible to differentiate the duration of fatigue into short (up to a week), medium (up to a month) and long (over a month), and to consider cancer more likely with medium- or long-term fatigue. However, this guide may be misleading, with the probable exception of isolated fatigue over 6 months in duration, which is unlikely to be malignant.

Box 4.3   Questions in a patient with fatigue

- How long has the fatigue been present?
- What other symptoms are present?

Box 4.4   Investigation of fatigue without other features

- Full blood count, plus ESR or CRP
- Thyroid function tests

What Other Symptoms are Present?

The differential diagnosis depends on both the duration of fatigue and the associated symptoms. As infections commonly cause short-term fatigue, the GP will initially focus on these. In a patient with medium- or long-term fatigue, the GP will have to consider autoimmune disorders, endocrine disease, chronic infections, alcoholism, sleep problems (such as sleep apnoea) or depression as likely diagnoses. In most cases, some clue to occult malignancy will emerge, and many of the above conditions can be eliminated from the differential diagnosis quite quickly.

Most GPs will take a full blood count when investigating fatigue. This may reveal anaemia, so raising the possibility of colorectal cancer, or a raised platelet count, hinting at lung cancer. It can be difficult to spot hypothyroidism clinically, so thyroid function testing seems appropriate. Obviously, any clues about disease in a particular organ should lead to focused investigation. Further investigation of fatigue aimed at uncovering cancer seems unnecessary, unless there are other symptoms in combination with the fatigue.

C-Reactive Protein and Erythrocyte Sedimentation Rate

These two tests are similar. They have specific uses: for instance, the ESR is useful in the diagnosis and monitoring of treatment for polymyalgia rheumatica, and CRP for some infections. However, in cancer diagnostics, the most common use is in the patient with vague symptoms, for which the GP is unable to find an explanation. The assumption is that the ESR or CRP will be raised when the patient has an organic disease such as cancer. The converse of this assumption is that the GP and patient can be reassured when the test is normal. The problem with these assumptions is that they have not been tested rigorously in primary care. Even in secondary care, the sensitivity of a very abnormal ESR (above 50 mm/hour) for cancer is around 50%, with a specificity of approximately 95%. The figures are unlikely to be as high in primary care. There are a few situations where the result is likely to be abnormal, such as disseminated cancer or with some haematological malignancies, particularly myeloma. Even so, most patients with disseminated cancer are clearly unwell and confirmation that they are ill by an abnormal ESR or CRP is not really much of a diagnostic advance. Equally, in most haematological malignancies the full blood count is clearly abnormal. In short, neither the ESR nor the CRP is of value as a diagnostic test for cancer in primary care.

Metastatic Disease

Most disseminated cancers spread locally first, and produce local symptoms. These symptoms are described in the individual chapters. However, there are two relatively common presentations of metastatic cancer that pose a diagnostic difficulty for GPs. The uncommon sites are, by definition, uncommon and little will be learned by reading a long list of atypical secondary sites.

These two presentations are of lymphadenopathy, in particular the isolated enlarged lymph node, and of bone pain. As usual, the difficulty is in deciding how likely malignancy is, and thus whether referral is warranted. This chapter deals with lymphadenopathy in adults; for children see Chapter 14.

The Isolated Lymph Node

A relatively common primary care scenario is the patient with a single swollen lymph node. This is usually in the neck, axilla or groin. As with all unexplained lumps, the patient (and doctor) will be concerned that the lump is a sign of cancer. This cancer could be a primary lymphoma, or a metastasis to the regional node from a primary elsewhere. Most research has focused on lymph nodes in the neck.

The Risk of Cancer in a Patient with an Isolated Lymph Node

Clearly the risk greatly depends on the duration of the lymphadenopathy and its properties on examination. If all patients with isolated lymphadenopathy are considered together, the risk of malignancy is 1% or less. An American study in primary care found no malignancies in 249 patients with isolated lymphadenopathy. In only 3% of patients was the lymphadenopathy even considered worrisome enough for a biopsy to be undertaken. Furthermore, in the majority of patients no final diagnosis was ever established. In a Dutch study, the only factors associated with cancer were older age and the gland or glands being in the neck. Neither of these studies described the nature of the lymphadenopathy, but it is safe to assume that hard or rubbery glands are associated with a higher risk of cancer. Indeed, that would presumably explain the very low rate of biopsy, in that soft glands were probably deemed worthy of watchful waiting in primary care rather than referral for biopsy.

The UK guidelines (2005 version) recommendations for urgent referral of lymphadenopathy, in the context of haematological cancer, are shown in Box 4.5.

How Long has the Node been Present?

The starting point is that very few nodes will prove to be cancer. The length of time that the node has been present will be very dependent on the patient's level of concern. Most malignant lymphadenopathy will be of relatively recent onset, although the same is true for lymphadenopathy secondary to infection. It is rare for chronic lymphadenopathy to be malignant, but some lymphomas can be very slow growing.

Is the Swelling Progressive?

This is fairly obvious. Although malignant lymphadenopathy may occasionally fluctuate, it is much more usually progressive. The choice of a 2 cm gland as worthy of urgent referral is somewhat arbitrary; glands associated with cancers may be smaller.

Box 4.5   UK guidelines (2005 version) recommendations for urgent referral of lymphadenopathy

- Lymphadenopathy persisting for 6 weeks or more (for neck glands the time scale is described as 'of recent onset'
- Lymph nodes increasing in size
- Lymph nodes greater than 2 cm
- Widespread lymphadenopathy
- Associated splenomegaly, night sweats or weight loss

Box 4.6   Questions in a patient with an isolated lymph node

- How long has the node been present?
- Is the swelling progressive?
- Have there been other unusual swellings or skin changes?
- What other symptoms are present?

Have there been Other Unusual Swellings or Skin Changes?

This is essentially a hunt for the site of a primary cancer. A secondary cancer in the neck will usually arise from a cancer above the diaphragm. Likely primaries are oral, laryngeal or lung cancer. Melanomas are a relatively common cause, and the primary lesion can regress spontaneously. In the axilla, the main concern is a primary breast cancer. In the groin, skin cancers of the legs or testicular or prostate cancers are the likeliest underlying cause.

What Other Symptoms are Present?

This is similar to the questioning described above for fatigue and weight loss. The GP is interested in identifying infections as a cause of the swollen lymph node.

Examination of the Patient with an Isolated Lymph Node

This depends on the site of the node, but is largely aimed at finding a primary tumour. A thorough examination is required, including of the mouth (oral cancer), chest (lung cancer) and abdomen (for masses, particularly an enlarged spleen). GPs are very good at deciding whether a lymph node may be malignant (even before reading this book). When GP referrals of unexplained lymphadenopathy are studied, 80–90% of malignant glands are referred within a month of first presentation to primary care. Equally importantly, 91–98% of benign glands are *not* referred.

The referral decision is easy if the nodes feel malignant. On palpation, they can be hard or 'craggy', suggesting a non-haematological cancer, or firm, which is more likely to be a lymphoma. A malignant node is rarely tender. If the node feels malignant, it is wisest to refer urgently for biopsy. There is little to be gained by a primary care hunt for the source of the cancer. However, few presentations with lymphadenopathy fall into this category. In patients in whom the lymphadenopathy is not obviously malignant, it is reasonable to organise a period of observation plus requesting the simple tests described below. In this instance the ESR may be helpful, as it may be significantly raised in haematological cancers.

Box 4.7   Investigation of lymphadenopathy without other features

- Full blood count, plus ESR or CRP
- CXR

Box 4.8   Questions in a patient with generalised lymphadenopathy

- How long have the nodes been present?
- What other symptoms are present, particularly of infection?

Generalised Lymphadenopathy

With generalised lymphadenopathy, there are fewer differential diagnoses, with malignancy and infection being the main possibilities. The size of the nodes is less important than with a single node. Nodes draining areas prone to multiple abrasions (perhaps associated with work or hobbies) or low-grade infections (such as those possibly associated with eczema) may be palpable, though they are rarely bigger than 1 cm. Children and adolescents have a greater lymphoid mass relative to their body weight, and often have palpable nodes that might be considered abnormal in an adult. As with isolated lymphadenopathy, it is important to identify any splenomegaly.

Most patients with generalised lymphadenopathy will require referral, unless there is a clear infective cause such as glandular fever. This infection is fairly easy to diagnose. In children, the Paul–Bunnell test may be negative, but a specific IgM antibody test for Epstein–Barr virus will be diagnostic. Much less commonly seen in UK practice is cytomegalovirus infection or HIV infection. Toxoplasmosis usually produces localised lymphadenopathy and mild non-specific 'viral' symptoms. Tests for toxoplasma IgG and IgM antibodies may be diagnostic of recent infection. All these tests can be analysed quickly and it is reasonable to delay referral while waiting for results, providing there is a good clinical reason to suspect infection. Otherwise, there is no point in delaying referral, nor in hunting for infection when it is not obvious.

Low-grade lymphoma and chronic lymphocytic leukaemia often present with generalised lymphadenopathy, but in Hodgkin's disease and high-grade lymphoma the disease is usually more localised. These are described further in Chapter 15.

The Possible Bone Metastasis

Most cancers can spread to bone, particularly breast, lung, prostate and thyroid. Some of the haematological cancers such as myeloma may have multiple deposits in the bone marrow (see Chapter 15). It is quite common for cancer to present with metastatic disease, rather than with symptoms from the primary. The main effects of bone secondaries are to cause pain, or to cause collapse of the bone in a pathological fracture. Investigation is generally easy, in that an X-ray will usually be diagnostic. In men, it is worth considering a PSA, as prostate cancer is the commonest cancer to spread to bone whilst the primary tumour is silent.

Malignant fractures can be very difficult to diagnose, as their onset may be gradual, and if the patient can tolerate the pain, loss of function may be gradual rather than dramatic. Malignant fracture of the hip is classically difficult to spot. However, once the possibility of a fracture has been considered, the X-rays will usually reveal that it is malignant in origin. Putting this more simply, the GP's role is to identify that a fracture has occurred; it is secondary care's responsibility to recognise it as malignant. Of course, the GP should be more aware of the possibility of a pathological fracture when their patient has a previous malignancy.

Malignant fractures of the vertebral column are a medical emergency. The onset is not necessarily rapid. Around half of patients have leg weakness for over 2 weeks before they are diagnosed. Patients with a longer duration of weakness also obtain much more benefit from radiotherapy than those with a rapid onset, presumably because in the latter, vertebral collapse and spinal cord compression are more severe. Three-quarters of patients have nerve root pain, leaving a quarter whose vertebral collapse is largely painless. As a diagnostic problem, malignant spinal cord compression is similar to other malignant fractures; the issue is for the GP to think of the diagnosis as a possible explanation of the symptoms. Once that is done, the investigation and management are largely done within secondary care.

Chapter 5

Breast Cancer

Clare Wilkinson

Epidemiology

Breast cancer is the most common new cancer overall in the UK, despite being almost entirely confined to women. There are over 41,000 new cases in the UK each year and GPs can expect to encounter one new case on average every 11 months. The annual incidence by age is shown in Figure 5.1. Despite increases in incidence, mortality from breast cancer in the UK has fallen since 1990 from 38/100,000 deaths to 32/100,000 in 2004. Breast cancer accounts for a third of all female cancers and women face an average lifetime risk of one in nine of developing the disease.

Three-quarters or more of breast cancers present symptomatically, as opposed to through a screening programme. Ten-year survival in women with node-negative disease approaches 80% and in node-positive women it is approximately 61%. General practitioners and other primary care professionals will care for a significant number of patients with breast cancer, at all stages from diagnosis to palliative care. Many survivors of breast cancer now have the equivalent of a chronic disease. Therefore, careful long-term management and surveillance are needed with well-organised physical and psychological care. This relates not just to detection of recurrence, but also to recognition and management of transient and long-lasting side-effects from treatment. This chapter will deal with various aspects of the primary care role, including timely diagnosis, management at various stages and issues of current importance to these women and their primary care teams.

Breast cancer causes over 21,000 deaths a year in the UK. Since many patients survive their cancer, prevalence is five times higher than this, with over 100,000 women living with the disease at any one time. Indeed, in the UK, while the incidence of breast cancer is increasing, survival has improved. The incidence itself varies fivefold across countries. Although this is predominantly a female cancer, men may also rarely develop the disease.

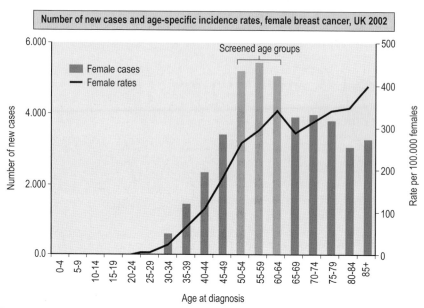

Figure 5.1   Number of new cases and age-specific incidence rates of breast cancer, UK 2002. Reproduced with permission from Cancer Research UK, Jan 2006. http://info.cancerresearchuk.org/cancerstats/types/breast/incidence/

The underlying cause of non-genetic breast cancer is unknown. The main risk factor is age. It is rare in women under 30, with risk doubling every 10 years until the menopause. Other risk factors include early age of menarche, late menopause and having fewer children. Those may all be related to the overall number of menstrual cycles a woman has had, with a higher number conferring more risk. Other risk factors include a family history of breast cancer, atypical hyperplasia, excess alcohol intake, obesity and use of hormone replacement therapy. Protection against breast cancer is conferred by having more children and by breastfeeding.

Mutations in the BRCA1 and BRCA2 genes are responsible for about 5% of breast cancers; these are strongly penetrant genes. Other less penetrant genes, including autosomal recessive genes, may be of aetiological importance in some families. Women with breast cancer are also at risk of a second contralateral cancer. This applies particularly to women with a family history and to women who have their first cancer at a younger age.

Presenting Symptoms

The usual presenting symptom of breast cancer is a lump, occurring in around 90% of women diagnosed outside mammography programmes.

> **Box 5.1   UK guidelines (2005 version) recommendations for urgent referral of possible breast cancer**
>
> - At any age, with a discrete hard lump with fixation, with or without tethering
> - At any age, with a previous cancer and a new lump or suspicious symptoms
> - Females of 30 years or older, with a discrete lump persisting after their next period or presenting after menopause
> - Females under 30, with an enlarging lump or one that is fixed and hard
> - At any age, with unilateral skin or nipple change resistant to topical treatment
> - With spontaneous nipple bleeding
> - Males over 50 with a unilateral breast lump

Some women may present with skin tethering, nipple changes or discharge or, in the case of inflammatory breast cancer, redness and swelling. Most women presenting with breast cancer will have primary operable disease, making early and timely diagnosis vital. Common sites of metastatic disease in women with either a late presentation or with a previous history of breast cancer include lung, causing breathlessness; bone, leading to pain or a pathological fracture; liver, with discomfort or nausea; or brain, presenting with seizures. The UK guidelines are summarised in Box 5.1.

Suspicion of malignancy should be high if the lump is hard, discrete, with fixation and with or without skin tethering. These signs should be treated as urgent irrespective of age. Lumps that persist between periods, or present after the menopause, should be regarded as suspicious. Patients who have unilateral bloody nipple discharge, those who have previously had breast cancer and present with a new lump and those with skin or nipple changes not responsive to topical treatments should also be urgently referred. It is not appropriate to undertake investigations in primary care prior to secondary care referral.

Clinical Examination

Most presentations occur when a woman has found a discrete lump in her breast. Breast tissue has a normal lumpiness; therefore, it is vital that GPs are familiar with normal breast tissue. Clinical examination involves checking both breasts, feeling with the flat of the fingers in each of four quadrants and under the nipple. Examination of the regional lymphatics should follow, especially the axilla and the supraclavicular nodes. If there is a suspicion of breast cancer, it is also wise to examine the respiratory system and the abdomen and to check for bony tenderness in the thoracic spine. Referral proformas incorporating national guidelines refined for local use should be available for all primary care teams to ensure timely appropriate referral to specialist breast teams.

Breast Problems with A Low Risk of Cancer

Most lumps in women under 30 years are benign and urgent referral of, for example, small clinical fibroadenomas is not appropriate. However, because breast cancer does rarely occur in this group, particular signs which should trigger suspicion include a lump that enlarges, that has other cancerous features or where there is concern regarding family history.

Patients with breast pain and no palpable abnormality do not require urgent referral and need only be referred at all if symptoms are severe or difficult to manage in primary care.

Minimising Diagnostic Delays

The essential message for GPs in terms of primary breast cancer is to refer lumps urgently and to ensure that correct systems are used to reach the cancer teams quickly. The essential message for minimising delay in identifying recurrences is to maintain an appropriate level of suspicion in women with a breast cancer history when presented with a new clinical symptom or sign.

Screening Programme and Breast Self-Examination

The UK NHS invites all women between the ages of 50 and 64 for a mammogram at 3-year intervals, as described in Chapter 3. Many of the abnormalities detected by screening prove to be ductal carcinoma in situ. This condition precedes invasive malignant stages. With ductal carcinoma in situ, the malignant cells have not broken through the basement membrane. Treatment is breast-conserving surgery followed by radiotherapy, sometimes supplemented with tamoxifen. The prognosis is excellent.

'Breast awareness' can be taught as knowing what your own breasts look like and feel like. Useful information to convey to women regarding breast awareness includes the following: they should report a new lump or thickening in the breast or armpit, changes in the skin such as dimpling, puckering or redness, changes in the nipple such as a change in the direction of the nipple or an unusual discharge, changes around the nipple such as an unusual rash or sore area or a change in the size or shape of the breast. It is worth reminding women, for the sake of reassurance, that nine out of 10 breast lumps are harmless and that all the signs listed here can have other causes. However, breast cancer is best treated early.

Breast-Self-Examination (BSE)

BSE is an intuitively attractive concept since, theoretically, a well-trained woman who practises BSE might improve her survival by detecting breast masses when they are relatively small. However, palpable breast masses are common and usually benign, particularly in young women. BSE may lead to unwarranted anxiety, false reassurance and unnecessary medical interventions. From the literature to date, BSE has not been shown to be effective in reducing breast cancer mortality.

Staging, Treatment and Recurrence

Although this book concentrates upon diagnosis, in breast cancer staging is particularly relevant as it determines the risk not only of death but also of recurrence. Although women are usually followed up by surgical teams, there is a move towards primary care follow-up, so GPs are increasingly involved in the diagnosis of recurrent disease. Of course, most recurrences are spotted by the woman herself, not by a doctor.

Early Operable Disease

Primary, operable breast cancer is defined as disease that is restricted to the breast and sometimes the local lymph nodes. This stage now has a very good prognosis, with many women achieving a cure. Women without nodal involvement have a 30–35% risk of recurrence within 5 years, compared with a 50–60% risk for node-positive women. Those with tumours larger than 4 cm are usually treated with mastectomy. Smaller tumours are usually treated with lumpectomy. Following surgery, most women in this category will also be treated with adjuvant radiotherapy, chemotherapy and tamoxifen.

Locally Advanced Disease

Locally advanced disease is defined as tumours that have spread to skin or chest wall or where axillary nodes are more heavily involved. This category includes stages TNM 3B and T4a–d. Recurrence is common and survival chances poorer. Treatment consists of surgery, sometimes with radiotherapy, followed by tamoxifen. There is little evidence that chemotherapy improves recurrence or survival rates.

Metastatic Disease

Metastatic breast cancer is currently considered incurable, but significant strides in survival have been made for this group over the last two decades. Even so, median survival is still only 2 years, although a few women may survive up to 15 years. The need for early diagnosis of recurrences is therefore an important message for GPs. The prognosis varies according to the woman's age, oestrogen receptor status and the extent of disease progression.

Follow-up Practices

Follow-up of women after breast cancer treatment is often carried out in secondary care settings on an annual basis, but few recurrences are diagnosed in this way. Most recurrences are presented as interval symptoms or signs. Women are at risk of recurrence for the rest of their lives, but most recurrences are detected in the first 5 years. Symptoms include changes in the breast or the chest wall, lymphadenopathy, weight loss, anaemia, persistent cough and/or unexplained musculoskeletal pain. Although these rather non-specific symptoms may frequently represent harmless conditions, around 75% of recurrences present in this way.

However, earlier detection of recurrence does not necessarily improve survival. Randomised trials studying intensive follow-up regimes compared to standard follow-up did not show any differences in overall survival. There is no evidence for the use of serum tumour markers to improve detection of recurrences.

Information needs of the other family members are also important. First-degree relatives of breast cancer patients often want information about their own risk of breast cancer, as well as information about risk factors and early detection measures. This is clearly a role for primary care. Women with a high-risk family history should be referred to a local cancer genetic clinic for consideration of genetic counselling and testing if they wish.

Current Issues in Breast Cancer

Sentinel node biopsy

Sentinel node biopsy is now widely used for staging breast cancer where there are no clinically palpable axillary nodes. It is a relatively simple procedure using imaging techniques to identify the first node in the lymphatic system draining a tumour site, thereby allowing this to be biopsied to assess nodal status rather than performing axillary clearance.

Tailoring Treatment to Individual Women

Significant advances have been made in the field of translational cancer research. These include genomics and proteomics, which continue to identify targets for anticancer treatments. Trastuzamab is a monoclonal antibody that is active against breast cancer in women who are positive for a specific receptor on the cancer cell and is the first biological agent to be approved for the treatment of metastatic breast cancer. Important issues still to be resolved include the best method for testing for HER2 status, the optimum schedule, dose and duration and the emergence of resistance. It is possible that in the near future women may have an optimal endocrine therapy sequence based on the genetic and molecular profile of individual tumours.

Further Reading/Key References

Bernard-Marty C, Cardoso F, Piccart M J 2004 Facts and controversies in systemic treatment of metastatic breast cancer. Oncologist 9:617–632

Burstein H J, Winer E P 2000 Primary care for survivors of breast cancer. New England Journal of Medicine 343:1086–1094

Chalmers K, Marles S, Tataryn D, Scott-Findlay S, Serfas K 2003 Reports of information and support needs of daughters and sisters of women with breast cancer. European Journal of Cancer Care 12:81–90

Chapter 6

Colorectal Cancer

William Hamilton

Epidemiology

Colorectal cancer is common, with over 34,000 new cases in the UK each year (Fig. 6.1). This equates to just less than six new diagnoses in a practice of 10,000 patients or around one new diagnosis per full-time GP. It is ranked third highest in male incidence (after prostate and lung), but is the second commonest new cancer in females (after breast). The incidence rose from the 1970s to the 1990s, but this increase has levelled off and there has been a small recent decrease. In contrast, mortality has declined slowly over the past 50 years.

The risk of colorectal cancer increases with age. A man aged over 85 has a 1 in 200 chance of developing colorectal cancer each year. This compares with a 1 in 500 chance for a man aged 65–69. Female figures are lower, with the same age groups having risks of 1 in 300 and 1 in 700, respectively. Although the risk for an individual rises continuously with age, the size of the total population at risk decreases. This balance between increasing risk and decreasing number of people at risk means that the number of new cases in each age group peaks at the age group 70–74 for both sexes. Half of new diagnoses are in patients aged 65–80.

Risk Factors

Familial Syndromes Including Colorectal Cancer

There are several inherited syndromes containing colorectal cancer as a feature, such as familial adenomatous polyposis, hereditary non-polyposis coli and Peutz–Jeghers syndrome. Familial adenomatous polyposis is the most common of these. It is autosomal dominant, so that someone with an

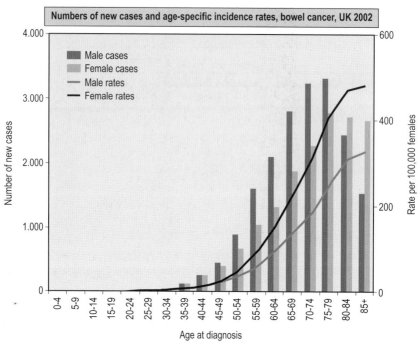

Figure 6.1   Annual incidence of colorectal cancer by age group (reproduced with permission from Cancer Research UK, Jan 2006. http://info.cancerresearchuk.org/ cancerstats/types/bowel/incidence/).

affected parent has a 50% chance of developing the condition themselves. The gene has been identified and reliable testing of individuals at risk can be now undertaken. In affected people, hundreds of adenomatous polyps develop in the colon during the teenage years. Transformation to cancer is almost inevitable by the age of 50, though it is usually earlier. Most patients elect to have a prophylactic colectomy.

The risks from hereditary non-polyposis coli and Peutz–Jeghers syndrome are lower than from familial adenomatous polyposis. They are usually managed by surveillance colonoscopies. Most cancers in families with these syndromes are identified in secondary care, so it is probable that the GP will have relatively little involvement in the management of such patients, other than identifying the family history in the first place. Should a cancer develop between rounds of surveillance colonoscopies, there is no reason to expect its presentation to be any different from colorectal cancers presenting in the general population, other than the patient being younger than the norm.

Family History of Colorectal Cancer

A familial predisposition to colorectal cancer is well recognised. In the general population, the lifetime risk of dying from colorectal cancer is approximately 1 in 50. This increases to 1 in 17 if any first-degree relative has had colorectal cancer and 1 in 10 if this relative was diagnosed below the age of 45. If two relatives develop cancer below the age of 45, then the risk of death from colorectal cancer is around 1 in 6. Twin studies estimate the inheritable component of the cancer to be around a third. However, no specific gene has been identified that accounts for the extra risk, other than the genes for the familial syndromes described above.

This contrasts with breast cancer, where a woman with a strong family history of cancer may choose to be tested for the BRCA gene; if her test is positive, she may consider prophylactic mastectomy. In colorectal cancer, such refinement of risk is not (yet) possible, so patients and their doctors need to decide if their adverse family history alone merits regular colonoscopy. Recent guidelines recommend colonoscopic surveillance of patients who have two first-degree relatives with colorectal cancer or one first-degree relative under 45 years. The first colonoscopy is recommended to be performed around the age of 35–40, with a second one at 55. The evidence for these recommendations is very indirect and such screening has not been taken up systematically. However, 4–7.5% of the healthy population have one first-degree relative with bowel cancer, so there is a large pool of people at higher risk, around 80–150 for each full-time GP. Such patients may well wish to discuss the possibility of surveillance. Many of these patients will be of the age group proposed for the national screening programme (see Chapter 3).

Inflammatory Bowel Disease

Ulcerative colitis and Crohn's disease both predispose to colorectal cancer. Around 1–2% of all colorectal cancers arise in patients with inflammatory bowel disease. The risk of a complicating cancer is similar for the two conditions and increases with the duration and extent of the inflammatory bowel disease. The diagnostic problem is that inflammatory bowel disease and colorectal cancer have similar symptoms: rectal bleeding, diarrhoea and sometimes fatigue, abdominal pain and anaemia. This can make identifying the complicating cancer difficult. For this reason, surveillance colonoscopies have been recommended, though again these recommendations are not based on firm research evidence. Current thinking is that surveillance colonoscopies should begin 8–10 years after disease onset for pancolitis and 15–20 years after the beginning of disease limited to the left side of the colon.

Diabetes

There is considerable epidemiological evidence for a link between diabetes and colorectal cancer. Cohort studies have estimated odds ratios of 1.6–1.8 for colorectal cancer in patients in the top quintile of blood sugar compared with those in the lowest quintile. These findings were simply on patients with above-average blood sugar levels, few of whom were actually diabetic. Slightly higher figures are found in patients who are diabetic, with odds ratios in the range 1.3–2.9. The link between diabetes and colorectal cancer probably relates to insulin-like growth factor 1 (IGF-1). IGF-1 competes for the same binding proteins in the plasma as insulin and is carcinogenic. When insulin levels are high (as in type II diabetes), more free IGF-1 is present in the circulation and thus its mitogenic effect is increased.

How can a GP use the fact that, in rough terms, diabetic patients have twice the risk of colorectal cancer than non-diabetics? The symptoms of colorectal cancer in a diabetic patient are likely to be the same as those experienced by others. Nonetheless, a GP should be slightly more willing to investigate diabetic patients with one of the symptoms described below. Fluctuations in weight and gastrointestinal disturbances are, however, common in diabetic patients without cancer. Referral may not therefore be required at the beginning of such symptoms, but early review in the practice is sensible.

Colorectal Cancer Presentation

There are three main pathways by which colorectal cancer is diagnosed. The first is asymptomatically, following a screening procedure. Around 5–20% of cancers are identified this way, with the highest figures from the US. With the steady increase in screening, the pattern of presentation is changing towards a higher proportion of asymptomatic cancers. Despite these changes, the large majority of patients with colorectal cancers in the UK present with symptoms to their GP and this is likely to continue to be the case for the foreseeable future.

Emergency Presentations

Some colorectal cancers present with surgical emergencies, principally obstruction or perforation; these account for 3–21% of hospital series, with UK figures among the highest. About half of adults with large bowel obstruction have an underlying cancer. Why the UK should have one of the highest rates of emergency presentation is not well understood. In part, it may represent British embarrassment at discussing bowel problems or a more general unwillingness to make a fuss with so-called 'minor' symptoms. It may not reflect the British character at all, but the rural nature of much of the UK. There is a close link between rurality and late-stage of the cancer at diagnosis. These may all equate to the same thing: the hill farmer in a far-flung outpost of Britain may be too embarrassed (or busy) to report symptoms; equally he or she may be too phlegmatic.

Mortality from emergency surgery has steadily improved over the last 20 years, mainly because of surgical and anaesthetic advances. Even so, it is clear that one of the main areas of potential improvement in colorectal cancer mortality is in a reduction of cases presenting as an emergency. Screening may do this: a small, but real, decrease in the proportion of patients presenting as an emergency was seen in the Nottingham study of screening using faecal occult bloods. Around 60% of patients who present with a bowel obstruction have experienced symptoms of colorectal cancer before the onset of the emergency. Indeed, in a recent UK audit of 154 cancers from three English cities, 39 had a surgical emergency. Ten of these occurred after their GP had referred them for investigation of suspected cancer, but before hospital investigations had been undertaken. If these patients (in whom colorectal cancer was obviously being considered) could have their emergency admission avoided, this should reduce overall mortality.

Symptomatic Presentation

Although some cancers are diagnosed through screening and some present as an emergency, most present to their GP with symptoms. The recent UK guidelines are summarised in Box 6.1.

Box 6.1   UK Guidelines (2005 version) Recommendations for Urgent Referral of Possible Colorectal Cancer

- Rectal bleeding with a change in bowel habit to looser stools and/or increased stool frequency persisting for 6 weeks or more (over 40s)
- Rectal bleeding without anal symptoms (such as soreness, discomfort, itching, lumps or prolapse) persisting for 6 weeks or more (over 60s)
- Change of bowel habit to looser stools and/or increased stool frequency, without rectal bleeding and persisting for 6 weeks or more (over 60s)
- A right lower abdominal mass (any age)
- A rectal mass (any age)
- Unexplained iron deficiency anaemia in men of any age (Hb below 11 g/dl) or non-menstruating women (Hb below 10 g/dl)

These symptoms may be present for a long time before diagnosis, even up to a year. There are five important symptoms: one or more of them is present in almost all patients with colorectal cancer (see Table 6.1). Indeed, 327 (94%) of 349 cases in the biggest primary care study from the UK had reported at least one of these symptoms to their GP in the year before diagnosis.

Rectal Bleeding

This is a classic symptom of colorectal cancer and probably the one most doctors would think of first. Around 40% of cases have reported rectal bleeding to their doctors in the year before the diagnosis is made. The risk of cancer has been estimated at between 2% and 7%. The risk rises with age, from 1.4% at ages 40–69 to 4.8% for patients aged 70 or above. This still means that the large majority of patients reporting rectal bleeding do not have cancer, whatever their age. The rise in risk from rectal bleeding with age is more than just the plain increase in risk with age. Two other factors are relevant: the proportion of colorectal cancers with rectal bleeding as a feature (which is roughly the same at all ages); and the frequency of rectal bleeding in the general population (which falls with age).

The above figures relate to rectal bleeding that has been reported to the doctor. This is only a small proportion of those who actually experience the symptom. In UK surveys, between 14% and 19% of the population describe rectal bleeding at some point in the last year. A first occurrence of bleeding is much rarer; around 2% of the population report their first ever episode of rectal bleeding in the previous year. This is summarised in Figure 6.2.

Table 6.1   The top five symptoms of colorectal cancer in primary care, along with the percentage of cases reporting this symptom to their GP before diagnosis and the positive predictive value of each symptom when presented in primary care

Symptom	Percentage of cases with this symptom before diagnosis	Percentage risk of colorectal cancer for a patient over 40 reporting this symptom to their GP
Rectal bleeding	42%	2–7
Diarrhoea	38%	0.94
Constipation	26%	0.42
Abdominal pain	42%	1.1
Weight loss	27%	1.2

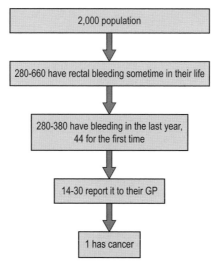

Figure 6.2 Incidence of rectal bleeding in the community and in primary care, presented for illustrative purposes for an assumed GP list size of 2000 patients (reproduced from Hamilton W, Sharp D 2004 Diagnosis of colorectal cancer in primary care: the evidence base for guidelines. Family Practice 21:99-104, by permission of Oxford University Press).

Box 6.2   Questions in a Patient with Rectal Bleeding

- How long has the bleeding been happening?
- What is the nature of the bleeding?
- What other symptoms are present?

Many patients do not report their bleeding as they consider themselves to have benign disease, usually haemorrhoids. Of course, given the small numbers of cancers, most of these patients are correct in assuming that their rectal bleeding is benign.

How Long has the Bleeding been Happening?

This question seeks to identify either new bleeding or recurrent spells of recent bleeding. There is little relationship between the actual duration of bleeding and the chance of the patient reporting it to their doctor. The risk of colorectal cancer is lower in patients who have had intermittent bleeding all their life, compared with those who are reporting a first spell, but is higher when the patient reports a recurrence of bleeding soon after the first episode. Having two episodes of rectal bleeding close together increases the risk to around 7%.

However, there is more to general practice than just manipulation of numbers and crude calculation of risk. The patient with rectal bleeding (or any other symptom of cancer) will have consulted for a reason. It is sensible to ask why they have chosen to report this episode of rectal bleeding. For a first spell of bleeding, the answer is likely to be obvious but for recurrences the patient will usually have identified something different or worrisome which has prompted them to consult. This may be nothing to do with colorectal cancer.

What is the Nature of the Bleeding?

This second question seeks to obtain a fuller description of the symptom, in particular the colour of the blood and whether it is mixed in with the stool.

The colour of the bleeding gives a clue as to the source: bright red, fresh blood is more likely to originate in the rectum and darker blood higher in the colon. This is not a completely reliable indicator, in that even cancer in the caecum can cause bright red bleeding. Blood mixed with the stool is more suggestive of cancer than blood coating the stool and dark blood mixed with the stool is particularly unfavourable, with a risk of cancer of over 10%.

What Other Symptoms are Present?

The risk of colorectal cancer posed by pairs of symptoms is shown in Figure 6.3. Having a second – or a third – symptom suggestive of colorectal cancer generally increases the risk of an underlying cancer. When diarrhoea accompanies rectal bleeding, the risk rises to 3.4% and when rectal bleeding occurs with loss of weight, the risk approaches 5%. However, the risk from rectal bleeding and constipation together is no higher than the risk for rectal bleeding alone. In part, this is because constipation is a very low-risk symptom; equally, it may be that straining with constipation increases the chance of rectal bleeding from haemorrhoids.

Box 6.3 Examination of a Patient with Rectal Bleeding

- Examine the abdomen, looking for masses
- Inspect for anaemia
- Do a rectal examination/proctoscopy

Risk of colorectal cancer for individual features, repeat presentations and for pairs of features (in the context of a background risk of 0.25%)

Constipation	Diarrhoea	Rectal bleeding	Loss of Weight	Abdominal pain	Abdominal tenderness	Abnormal rectal exam	Haemoglobin 10–13g/dl	Haemoglobin 10 g/dl	
0.42	0.94	2.4	1.2	1.1	1.1	1.5	0.97	2.3	Risk as a single symptom
0.81	1.1	2.4	3.0	1.5	1.7	2.6	1.2	2.6	Constipation
	1.5	3.4	3.1	1.0	2.4	11	2.2	2.9	Diarrhoea
		6.8	4.7	3.1	4.5	8.5	3.6	3.2	Rectal bleeding
			1.4	3.4	6.4	7.4	1.3	4.7	Loss of weight
				3.0	1.4	3.3	2.2	6.9	Abdominal pain
					1.7	5.8	2.7	>10	Abdominal tenderness

Figure 6.3 Risk of colorectal cancer for individual features, repeat presentations and for pairs of features (in the context of a background risk of 0.25%) (adapted from Hamilton et al 2005).

Examine the Abdomen, Looking for Masses

Around 5% of colorectal cancers have a palpable abdominal mass. This equates to one cancer diagnosable by abdominal examination over a GP's clinical lifetime. A lot of abdomens will have to be palpated just to identify this one patient.

Examine for Anaemia

Clinical diagnosis of anaemia is supposed to be very difficult. Nonetheless, inspection of the sclerae takes very little time and probably acts as a reminder to measure the haemoglobin. Severe anaemia is not that hard to identify clinically, as long as the GP thinks to look. As well as clinical examination for anaemia, the GP must decide whether to measure the haemoglobin when a patient describes rectal bleeding. As can be seen from Figure 6.3, even mild anaemia increases the risk of cancer to over 3%. There is an argument for measuring the haemoglobin in every patient with rectal bleeding, other than those with a clear cause, such as haemorrhoids.

Examine the Anus and do a Rectal Examination

The most useful examination is a rectal examination, which can be supplemented by a proctoscopy. Between a quarter and a half of rectal carcinomas are palpable on rectal examination. Of colorectal cancers as a whole, around 15% are palpable rectally. Most GPs can perform proctoscopy, which is useful not only for visualising any rectal mass but for identifying haemorrhoids. In theory, haemorrhoids and colorectal cancers can co-exist; in practice, haemorrhoids are the likeliest cause of uncomplicated rectal bleeding or bleeding with local anal symptoms.

Change in Bowel Habit

No patient ever comes into the surgery complaining of change in bowel habit. They complain of constipation or diarrhoea or sometimes both. Indeed, when used in the UK, the phrase has connotations of suspected colorectal cancer over and above its literal meaning. When GPs write in the notes 'change of bowel habit', they are really writing, 'change of bowel habit and I think colorectal cancer is a possibility'.

Diarrhoea

This is almost as common as rectal bleeding, with around 40% of patients reporting it to their doctors before diagnosis. The word 'diarrhoea' encompasses two different phenomena, though they can occur together. It can mean more frequent stools or looser stools. It may also co-exist with constipation; indeed, alternating constipation and diarrhoea may be a particular marker for malignancy.

Like rectal bleeding and constipation, diarrhoea is very common in the general population. Nearly a quarter of people report some urgency of defaecation and 1 in 10 has loose stools frequently. Most patients wait to see if their diarrhoea will settle before making an appointment with their doctor. Indeed, in those who have a cancer, the average duration of diarrhoea before the patient consults their GP is nearly 10 weeks. In one way this delay is

---

Box 6.4 Questions in a Patient with Change in Bowel Habit

- Is it constipation or diarrhoea or both?
- How long has it been present?

helpful, as the UK guidelines suggest referral if a patient has diarrhoea of 6 weeks' duration (or rectal bleeding plus diarrhoea of any duration). Patients allowing themselves time for the diarrhoea to settle means that most have had their symptom long enough at their first presentation to the doctor to qualify for urgent referral.*

Diarrhoea is the cancer symptom with the longest doctor delay (timed from first presentation to referral). Why should this be so? The simple answer is that an isolated complaint of diarrhoea truly is a low risk for cancer; approximately one in 200 patients aged between 40 and 70 years complaining of diarrhoea will have cancer. Even in patients over 70, only one patient in 70 will have cancer. Furthermore, around 5% of people over the age of 40 complain to their GP of diarrhoea each year. So, GPs see patients with diarrhoea frequently, yet only see one colorectal cancer a year. They cannot investigate for cancer in every patient with diarrhoea. Luckily, there are some additional features that can help to distinguish the few with cancer from the many without. These are summarised in Box 6.5.

Other Symptoms Together with Diarrhoea

Having a second symptom as well as diarrhoea increases the risk of cancer, even the so-called 'low-risk' symptom of constipation. The risk from combinations of symptoms is shown in Figure 6.3. One potential error is to ascribe any accompanying weight loss to the loss of appetite that is common with gastrointestinal disturbances. The risk from combined weight loss and diarrhoea – 1 in 30 – is probably high enough on its own to require investigation.

> ### Box 6.5   Features of Diarrhoea Particularly Suspicious for Cancer
>
> - Diarrhoea accompanied by one of the other four symptoms (rectal bleeding, abdominal pain, weight loss or constipation)
> - A second (or third) consultation with the patient still complaining of diarrhoea
> - Blood noted on microscopy of a stool specimen

---

*This makes the naive assumption that doctors obey guidelines. They don't, with an important proportion of patients fulfilling the criteria for urgent referral not receiving one and, conversely, several patients being sent for urgent referral who do not meet the criteria. This would be lamentable, apart from the crucial point that some of those patients who do not meet the criteria actually do have cancer, which the GP has picked up using "clinical acumen". It cannot be said too often that guidance (regrettably, including this book) is only guidance, not chapter and verse. Sometimes, doctor does know best . . .

A Second Consultation with Diarrhoea

This is a particular marker for cancer, though, as always, there are several alternative possibilities. A fair approximation is that each time the patient attends their GP complaining of diarrhoea, their risk of colorectal cancer doubles. This may simply represent that the diarrhoea has persisted (in itself a worrying feature) or that the patient is especially concerned (an even more worrying feature). This may be one of the examples of the patient knowing best; if they think 'something must be wrong' then perhaps something is. Under these circumstances, a full exploration of the problem is warranted. This includes abdominal and rectal examination and checking a stool sample and haemoglobin.

Blood Noted on Microscopy of a Stool Specimen

Most GPs will request microscopy and culture of a stool sample for patients with persistent diarrhoea. The primary purpose of microscopy is to identify parasites. However, red blood cells may be observed in the stool, without any other abnormal microscopy findings. This is an important marker for colorectal cancer. A patient with diarrhoea and a negative stool culture, but with red blood cells noted on their stool sample, is at high risk for cancer.

Constipation

If diarrhoea is a tricky subject for the GP, constipation is worse. It is a common symptom in those with colorectal cancer, about a quarter of patients having it. It is also very common in the general population. Up to a quarter of the UK population say that they have to strain to pass a stool and 14% describe themselves as constipated. Around 5–10% of the population will report constipation to their GP in any one year. Worse still, constipation is much more common in right-sided bowel cancer than left-sided cancer, so a tumour is unlikely to be palpable rectally. How can the GP identify the one underlying cancer among all these patients complaining of constipation?

Other Symptoms Together with Constipation

Colorectal cancer will not be the first diagnosis that a GP thinks of when their patient is constipated. Rightly so, as the risk is less than 1 in 200. It may be a side-effect of some drugs (particularly opiate analgesics, anti-cholinergics, antidepressants and antispasmodics, though almost any drug can be implicated). Dietary change can cause constipation, especially in the

> **Box 6.6   Features of Constipation Particularly Suspicious for Cancer**
>
> - Constipation accompanied by other symptoms (rectal bleeding, abdominal pain, weight loss or diarrhoea)
> - A second consultation with the patient still complaining of constipation
> - No alternative diagnosis, such as medication side-effects

elderly, whose fibre intake may fall. It can follow ill health of any cause. Particularly difficult in terms of identifying possible cancer is the constipation that can follow a spell of infectious diarrhoea. In many patients, there is no apparent cause. Constipation without other symptoms is very unlikely to represent an underlying cancer.

A Second (or third) Consultation with Constipation

In a similar way to diarrhoea, the risk of the patient having an underlying cancer to account for their symptom rises each time they report constipation to their doctor. It starts from a lower level of risk, at 0.4% for the first episode. Again, like diarrhoea, the risk roughly doubles with each presentation, so that by the third presentation it is well over 1%. Of course, this is still quite low.

No Alternative Explanation for the Constipation

Although many patients with constipation never have a cause identified, dietary changes and medication side-effects account for the majority. Most of these patients will be helped by treatment of the cause, perhaps with laxatives as well. In the remaining group, with no identifiable cause and who may well re-consult, colorectal cancer should at least be considered. Full examination, including a rectal, is appropriate, as well as checking the haemoglobin and a faecal occult blood. These latter two tests may be the only clues to identifying the right-sided tumour that sometimes causes constipation.

Abdominal Pain

Abdominal pain is extremely prevalent in the general population. It is less common in the elderly. This may not reflect a true lower incidence of pain but simply that the elderly have experienced intermittent pain for years and regard it as part of normal life rather than a symptom requiring attention and/or reporting to their GP. As with rectal bleeding, the patient's decision to consult their doctor depends on whether they perceive the symptom as a health problem or not. Roughly a quarter of those with pain do consult and most of these have a self-limited illness for which no definitive diagnosis can be found. Only 0.4–1.0% of primary care patients attending their doctor complaining of abdominal pain will have a diagnosis of colorectal cancer established within the next year.

What is the Nature of the Abdominal Pain?

This question is aimed at identifying other (more common) causes of abdominal pain. Many of the alternative diagnoses, such as dyspepsia or biliary or renal pain, are reasonably easy to identify. It is the vague, inexplicable abdominal pain that can signify cancer. Such a pain can be present for many months before a cancer is diagnosed – or even suspected.

As well as the non-specific pain that can be present for many months, incipient obstruction can present with colicky abdominal pain. This can precede the emergency admission by several weeks. It can be tempting to label this as 'colic' or irritable bowel syndrome. No doubt both exist but in 8% of UK patients with colorectal cancer, a diagnosis of irritable bowel syndrome was given during the year before the cancer was identified. If you believe your elderly patient has irritable bowel syndrome, then it would be wise to review them to ensure that the diagnosis is correct.

A Second (or third) Consultation with Abdominal Pain

Constipation, diarrhoea and abdominal pain have several non-malignant causes. Many of these causes are easily detected and treated in primary care. Therefore, it should not be surprising that repeat attendances with abdominal pain – which will be more likely when the condition has not been diagnosed – increase the chance that the patient has colorectal cancer. As with constipation and diarrhoea, the risk approximately doubles with each attendance for abdominal pain.

Box 6.7   Questions in a Patient with Abdominal Pain

- What is the nature of the pain?
- How often has the patient complained of it?
- How long has this pain been present?
- What other symptoms are present?

How Long has the Pain been Present?

This is similar to the issue of repeat attendances, in that both represent continued symptoms. Figure 6.4 shows primary care attendances by patients complaining of abdominal pain in those patients who were ultimately diagnosed with colorectal cancer (dark line), compared with controls of the same age and sex (light line). The rates of reporting abdominal pain separate somewhere between 6 months and a year before diagnosis, but they diverge much more widely from a point in time 6 months before diagnosis. Thus, any abdominal pain that the patient has had for over a year is extremely unlikely to be due to a colorectal cancer. If the pain has been present for 6 months to a year, the risk is still very small.

What Other Symptoms are Present?

As with all the five main symptoms, the risk of cancer is higher when a second symptom is present. For these 'softer' symptoms like abdominal pain, it is important to ask about all five symptoms.

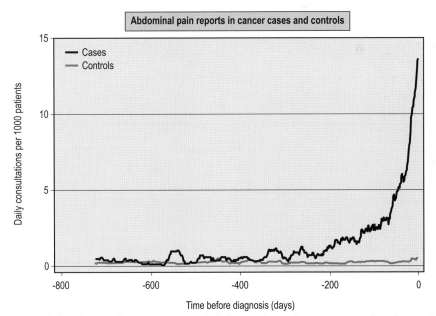

Figure 6.4 Timescale of reporting of abdominal pain by patients with colorectal cancer (adapted from Hamilton et al 2005).

Other Ways in which Colorectal Cancer may Present to Primary Care

Local Anal Symptoms

Symptoms such as pain on defaecation, tenesmus and pruritus can be a feature of rectal cancer. They are also very common in the general population, although their precise frequencies are unknown; hence the exact risk of cancer is also unknown but is probably quite low. One pitfall particularly applies to haemorrhoids. These can bleed and if examination of a patient complaining of rectal bleeding reveals a haemorrhoid, it is usually correct to ascribe the bleeding to the haemorrhoid. In most cases this will be right but it is wise to consider the (small) possibility of a cancer too. Treatment can be targeted at the haemorrhoid initially but should the patient experience further bleeding, investigation is warranted.

Iron Deficiency Anaemia

Iron deficiency anaemia is a classic pointer to colorectal cancer. It is present in 11–57% of patients with colorectal cancer and is particularly suggestive of caecal tumours. It generally signifies an underlying illness, so would normally be investigated as a matter of course.** In the general population, the prevalence of anaemia increases with age. Using a threshold of 13.0 g/dl in men and 12.0 g/dl in women, 4.4% of men and 6.6% of women aged 50–64 years are anaemic. Anaemia becomes progressively more common with increasing age. In those over 85 years, 26% of men and 20% of women are anaemic.

Colorectal cancer is one of the initial differential diagnoses but may not be the most likely cause. Inadequate dietary iron is common in the elderly, as is the anaemia of chronic disease. General practice studies suggest that around 10% of patients over the age of 40 with iron deficiency anaemia have colorectal cancer as the cause. Investigation for gastrointestinal blood loss in a patient with iron deficiency anaemia is therefore mandatory. However, only half of patients are adequately investigated for possible gastrointestinal blood loss.

** Blood test results do not just appear out of thin air. Someone, somewhere, has decided to test the haemoglobin. This is relevant, as almost all research papers on iron deficiency anaemia start from the abnormal blood test. In general practice, the blood should have been taken for a reason and so the significance of the abnormal result has to be considered in conjunction with the reason for testing.

Faecal Occult Bloods

Faecal occult blood testing is used in two main ways. The first is for screening, as described in Chapter 3. The second is in the investigation of possible gastrointestinal bleeding. A positive result in a faecal occult test mandates investigation of the bowel to identify the site of the bleeding. In primary care patients with lower gastrointestinal symptoms, around 1 in 10 of those with a positive faecal occult blood will have a colorectal cancer.

Further Reading/Key References

Andrieu N, Launoy G, Guillois R, Ory-Paoletti C, Gignoux M 2004 Estimation of the familial relative risk of cancer by site from a French population based family study on colorectal cancer (CCREF study). Gut 53:1322–1328

Cade D, Selvachandran S, Hodder R, Ballal M 2002 Prediction of colorectal cancer by consultation questionnaire. Lancet 360:278–283

Dunlop M 2002 Guidance on large bowel surveillance for people with two first degree relatives with colorectal cancer or one first degree relative diagnosed with colorectal cancer under 45 years. Gut 51 (suppl V):v17–v20

Hamilton W, Sharp D 2004 Diagnosis of colorectal cancer in primary care: the evidence base for guidelines. Family Practice 21:99–106

Hamilton W, Round A, Sharp D, Peters T 2005 Clinical features of colorectal cancer before diagnosis: a population-based case-control study. British Journal of Cancer 93:399–405

Hardcastle J D, Chamberlain J O, Robinson M H et al 1996 Randomised controlled trial of faecal-occult-blood screening for colorectal cancer. Lancet 348:1472–1477

Chapter 7

Lung Cancer
Christine Campbell and David Weller

Epidemiology

Lung cancer is the most common cause of cancer death in the world, with around 38,400 new cases in the UK each year. One in seven new cancers is a lung cancer, making it the second most frequently diagnosed cancer after breast cancer. In a general practice of 10,000 patients, around 6–7 new diagnoses will be made each year. It is more common in men than women, although the male rate is falling and the female rate increasing, reflecting recent changes in smoking in women.

As with most cancers, lung cancer risk increases with age. It is rare under the age of 40 but increases markedly with age, peaking at 70–79 years (Fig. 7.1). It is the commonest cause of cancer death in both men and women with approximately 36,000 deaths in 2002 in the UK; indeed, survival rates for lung cancer are very poor compared with other cancers. One-year survival in the UK is approximately 25% and 5-year survival between 5% and 7%, with little improvement since the 1970s. Survival rates are higher in many European countries and in the US, possibly due to differences in treatment practice and stage at presentation.

Deprivation and Geographical Variation

Unlike most common cancers, the incidence of lung cancer has a clear association with lower socio-economic status in the UK, with a two- to three-fold difference between higher and lower socioeconomic groups. These differences are largely related to smoking. The highest incidence rates are in Scotland and in England there is a clear 'North-South' divide.

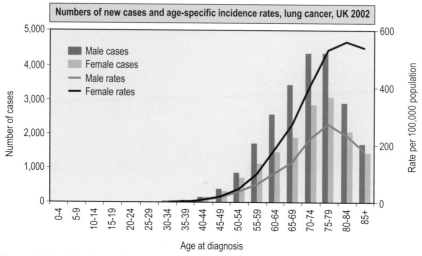

Figure 7.1   Number of new cases and age-specific annual incidence rates of lung cancer by sex, UK 2002 (reproduced with permission from Cancer Research UK, Jan 2006. http://info.cancerresearchuk.org/cancerstats/types/lung/incidence/).

Risk Factors for Lung Cancer

GPs face considerable challenges in making a diagnosis of lung cancer. The symptoms are often quite non-specific and can be attributable to many other, more common causes. It is therefore important to identify predisposing factors to lung cancer, the most important being smoking.

Smoking

With tobacco also implicated in the development of numerous other cancers, smoking is by far the greatest risk factor for lung cancer, being associated with 90% of cases. The risk of developing lung cancer increases with the duration of smoking, the level of consumption and the tar content of the cigarettes.

Cigarette smoking became popular among men in the UK in the early 20th century, reaching a peak in the mid 1940s when 65% of men smoked. The prevalence of smoking among men has declined since 1974; in 2002, 27% of those aged 16 years and over smoked. Among women, just over 40% smoked in the 1950s and 1960s; that figure had decreased to 25% by 2002. Nonetheless, approximately 1 in 4 adults in the UK still smokes and health promotion will continue to be a major part of lung cancer prevention strategies.

Smoking in Young People

Around 450 children start smoking each day in the UK. By the age of 15 years, as many as 1 in 4 regularly smokes (defined as *at least* one cigarette each week). Rates are higher among girls than boys (26% versus 20%), although boys smoke more heavily than girls.

Smoking Cessation

Primary care has an important role in providing guidance and support to patients regarding stopping smoking: there is evidence that GPs can reduce smoking rates by providing appropriate advice. It is important to emphasise to patients the considerable health benefits of smoking cessation even for people who have smoked for many years. In men, the cumulative risk of dying from lung cancer by the age of 75 in life-long smokers falls from 16% to 10% for those who stop smoking at 60 and to 6% for those who stop at 50. In women the equivalent figures are a reduction from 10% to 5% and 2%. NICE has recommended the use of bupropion and nicotine replacement therapy for smokers who wish to stop.

Environmental Tobacco Smoke

It is now well accepted that exposure to environmental tobacco smoke (or passive smoking) increases the risk of lung cancer in adult non-smokers. Non-smokers living with a smoker have an estimated 24% greater risk of lung cancer and this risk is directly related to both the number of cigarettes and the years of exposure. Non-smokers exposed to tobacco in the workplace have an increased risk estimated to be 16–19%. Overall, about a quarter of lung cancers in never-smokers can be attributed to exposure to passive smoking.

Family History

The precise role of inherited susceptibility to lung cancer is unclear. Only a relatively small proportion of those who smoke develop lung cancer, leading to the hypothesis that individuals differ in their genetic susceptibility to the disease. A family history of lung cancer gives an independent, increased risk of lung cancer (even when smoking is controlled for) with the genetic component of lung cancer estimated to be 14%.

A candidate lung cancer predisposition gene has been reported, leading to the possibility of the future identification of causal genetic mutations. There are also some rare familial syndromes associated with lung cancer, including xeroderma pigmentosum, Bloom's, Werner's and Li-Fraumeni's syndromes. Increased rates of lung cancer have been reported in carriers of retinoblastoma gene mutations.

Other Risk Factors

More than any other cancer, lung cancer is related to occupational carcinogen exposure, with 9–15% of cancers having such exposure as a contributory factor. Although the contribution of occupational exposure to the development of lung cancer is small compared to that of cigarette smoking, it is large compared to most other risk factors. Tar, soot, arsenic, chromium, polycyclic hydrocarbons and nickel have all been identified as risk factors.

Asbestos exposure is strongly linked to lung cancer (as well as to mesothelioma), with a dose–response relationship. The peak incidence is 30–35 years following the initial exposure to asbestos. Although regulations have been in place in the UK for several decades to protect workers against asbestos dust, asbestos-related lung cancers still occur in older men in some areas of the UK. Mesotheliomas are also on the increase, with the peak expected early in the 2010s and a slow decline thereafter.

Radon is a naturally occurring carcinogen and uranium workers with high levels of exposure had an increased risk of lung cancer. Up to 5% of lung cancers in England and Wales have been attributed to residential radon exposure.

Chronic obstructive pulmonary disease (COPD) is associated with the development of lung cancer. Patients with COPD have a 4–6-fold increased risk of lung cancer, independent of their smoking history. Although there is continuing debate regarding the biological mechanism that accounts for this association, the presence of COPD is a useful clinical indicator of an increased risk of lung cancer.

Types of Lung Cancer

The major histological subtypes of invasive lung cancer (all of which are linked with cigarette smoking) include squamous cell carcinomas (around 35–45%), adenocarcinomas (about 15%) and large cell carcinomas (about 10%). These three are usually grouped into the non-small cell carcinomas (NSCLC), comprising approximately 75% of diagnoses. Small cell carcinomas (SCLC) account for 25% of diagnoses. As treatment options differ across these subtypes, it is essential that a histological diagnosis is made.

Staging

The TNM staging system, based on the characteristics of the primary tumour (location, size, invasion of adjacent structures), the regional lymph nodes and metastatic involvement, is used in the classification of NSCLC and stage assigned on the basis of these categories. Although the 5-year survival for stage I NSCLC patients treated with radical surgery is over 60% (and can be as high as 80% for very early squamous cell carcinomas), most patients with NSCLC present with advanced disease when curative treatment is not longer possible.

A two-stage classification system is generally used for SCLC tumours: they are classed as either 'limited' or 'extensive', depending on the extent to which the cancer has spread. 'Limited' refers to tumours that are confined to one lung and to the lymph nodes on the same side of the chest; 'extensive' refers to those cases where the disease has spread to both lungs, to lymph nodes on the other side of the chest or to other organs, including pleural fluid. Approximately 30% of patients present with limited and 70% with extensive disease. SCLC tumours usually progress rapidly and survival with untreated disease is on average less than 3 months. Radical surgery is rarely an option; chemotherapy and radiotherapy are used both to extend life expectancy and in palliation.

Potential Markers

A series of genetic and molecular changes have been identified in lung cancers and premalignant lesions, theoretically offering identifiable molecular biomarkers from blood, exhaled air or sputum. Circulating tumour-derived DNA is elevated in lung cancer patients compared to controls, suggesting its possible use as a diagnostic marker. Ultimately, it is hoped to develop a blood test that can detect premalignant changes or early-stage disease. Similarly, raised biomarkers in the exhaled breath of lung cancer patients compared to controls suggest their potential applicability as screening or diagnostic tests. DNA-based assays to detect abnormal DNA in sputum are also being investigated. It will, of course, be important to validate the predictive values of these and other potential molecular biomarkers extensively before they are investigated in large-scale trials. Their clinical utility in primary care is therefore still a number of years away.

Symptomatic Presentation

Eighty to ninety percent of lung cancer patients in the UK are diagnosed following presentation to primary care, with the next commonest route to diagnosis being via Accident and Emergency. However, those first presenting to primary care may not be identified as having lung cancer; in one recent study, 70 different pathways of referral to the final consultant were identified.

Early Detection Based on Symptoms

In common with many other cancers, the symptoms of lung cancer pose significant diagnostic challenges. It is very difficult to distinguish between those respiratory symptoms that carry increased risk of lung cancer and those that do not. The symptoms of lung cancer, such as cough, haemoptysis and weight loss, are common in primary care and the average GP will see less than two new lung cancers per year. Additionally, a large number of symptoms are experienced by patients in the months prior to diagnosis and they are frequently non-specific. Unlike other cancers, there are rarely significant delays between the onset of symptoms and presentation to a GP; it is generally in the region of 3 weeks. Furthermore, GPs are usually quick to investigate, usually with a chest X-ray.

The UK NICE guidelines relating to possible lung cancer are summarised in Box 7.1. These recommend that patients presenting with symptoms suggestive of lung cancer should be referred to a team specialising in the management of lung cancer. This has been shown to improve outcome: a large study in Scotland demonstrated increased survival at both 1 year (24.4% versus 11.1%) and 3 years (8.1% versus 3.7%) in patients who saw a respiratory physician.

There are some differences between the 2005 NICE guidelines and those issued by the Scottish Executive and the Scottish Intercollegiate Network Guidelines. The latter guidelines recommend referral for a chest X-ray in the case of unexplained or persistent fatigue in a smoker aged over 50 years, and urgent referral to a lung cancer specialist when any suspicious symptoms persist for 6 weeks or longer, even if the chest X-ray is normal.

To guide decision making, it is important to attempt to attach predictive values to symptoms and groups of symptoms. A recent study in the UK has produced such statistics and Figure 7.2 shows the PPVs for lung cancer for individual risk markers and pairs of risk markers in combination. The top row gives the positive predictive value (PPV) as a percentage for an individual symptom. The cells along the diagonal relate to the PPV when the same feature has been reported twice. Thus the cough/cough intersect is the PPV for lung cancer when a patient has attended twice (or more often) with cough. Other cells show the PPV when a patient has two different features.

Haemoptysis

Haemoptysis is an alarming symptom for patients. There are several common benign causes for this symptom, including chest infections; if such a cause is obviously present, it is reasonable for the GP to defer investigation.

Box 7.1   UK guidelines (2005 version) recommendations for possible lung cancer

Immediate referral to hospital
- Superior vena caval obstruction (swelling of the face and/or neck with fixed elevation of jugular venous pressure)
- Stridor

Urgent referral to respiratory specialist
- Persistent haemoptysis in smokers or ex-smokers aged 40 years or older
- Chest X-ray suggestive of lung cancer (including pleural effusion and slowly resolving consolidation)

Urgent referral for a chest X-ray
- Haemoptysis
- Unexplained, persistent (>3 weeks' duration):
  - chest and/or shoulder pain
  - dyspnoea
  - weight loss
  - chest signs
  - hoarseness
  - finger clubbing
  - cervical and/or supraclavicular lymphadenopathy
  - cough with or without any of the above
  - features suggestive of metastasis from lung cancer

Consideration of urgent referral for a chest X-ray or to a lung cancer specialist team
Any of the above signs and symptoms even if duration is less than 3 weeks in patients in high-risk groups:
- current or ex-smokers
- those with COPD
- those who have had asbestos exposure
- those with a previous cancer diagnosis

Nevertheless, haemoptysis is an important marker for lung cancer; it is reported by 20–40% of cases (but by 1.5% patients without cancer over a 2-year period) and 3% of patients report it as a first symptom.

Figure 7.2 shows that the PPV of haemoptysis is 2.4%, rising to 17% for a second presentation. Importantly, the risk of cancer is higher with the following additional symptoms: fatigue, dyspnoea, chest pain, loss of appetite and loss of weight. If a patient presents with haemoptysis

Risk of lung cancer for individual features, repeat presentations and for pairs of features

Cough	Fatigue	Dyspnoea	Chest pain	Loss of weight	Loss of appetite	Thrombo-cystosis	Abnormal spirometry	Haemoptysis	
0.40	0.43	0.66	0.82	1.1	0.87	1.6	1.6	2.4	PPV as a single symptom
0.58	0.63	0.79	0.76	1.8	1.6	2.0	1.2	2.0	Cough
	0.57	0.89	0.84	1.0	1.2	1.8	4.0	3.3	Fatigue
		0.88	1.2	2.0	2.0	2.0	2.3	4.9	Dyspnoea
			0.95	1.8	1.8	2.0	1.4	5.0	Chest pain
				1.2	2.3	6.1	1.5	9.2	Loss of weight
					1.7	0.9	2.7	>10	Loss of appetite
							3.6	>10	Thrombocytosis
								>10	Abnormal spirometry
								17	Haemoptysis

Figure 7.2 Risk of lung cancer for individual features, repeat presentations and for pairs of features (adapted from Hamilton et al 2005, by permission of BMJ Publishing Group).

plus any of these symptoms, an urgent chest X-ray is warranted. Even with a negative chest X-ray, referral to a respiratory specialist is wise as cancer can be present despite a negative chest X-ray. The combination of haemoptysis and cough has a lower PPV than haemoptysis alone; in a chest infection, cough may be accompanied by haemoptysis. Should the symptom persist without an obvious alternative diagnosis, it is an indication for referral.

Weight Loss and Fatigue

These are common symptoms in lung cancer and are discussed in Chapter 4. Weight loss is not necessarily a marker of end-stage disease, in that it can frequently be associated with operable disease.

Cough

Again, this is a very common symptom in the general population. One survey in the UK identified cough as having a prevalence of over 20%; another estimated that 52% of requests to pharmacists regarding symptoms are about respiratory problems, including cough. Similarly in general practice – cough is the most common symptom seen in primary care. Chronic cough is present in over 50% of those who smoke and, while most commonly associated with COPD, it is also a feature of lung cancer. In primary care, cough is a symptom of lung cancer in a quarter to two-thirds of patients (reported rates vary depending on the study design and population).

Although cough is common with lung cancer, lung cancer is uncommon with cough. Even with a chronic cough, the risk is less than 2%. As shown in Figure 7.2, the PPV for cough on first presentation is low and stays low on subsequent consultations, even when combined with any of the other common symptoms. Nonetheless, for many patients diagnosed with lung cancer, cough is the first symptom that prompts them to seek medical advice. If smokers describe a new cough or a change in a pre-existing cough, lung cancer should be considered. In the presence of subtle changes in a chronic cough or any unexplained cough that persists, investigation by chest X-ray is generally warranted and consideration should be given to referral even if the chest X-ray is negative.

Dyspnoea

While this is an important feature of presentation in lung cancer, it is more commonly found in other conditions such as heart failure. Dyspnoea without other symptoms is very rarely due to lung cancer (see Fig. 7.2).

However, when present with other symptoms, notably haemoptysis, the PPV is much higher, warranting investigation. A chest X-ray should be performed in all cases of unexplained or persistent dyspnoea, since it helps the identification of the more common causes as well as any cancer.

Chest Pain

This is usually a symptom of advanced lung cancer and indicates a poor prognosis. Like dyspnoea, chest pain rarely occurs as a solitary symptom. In general, investigation will focus initially on cardiac and/or musculoskeletal conditions. Unexplained shoulder pain may also warrant further investigation, looking for the (rare) Pancoast tumour.

Hoarseness

Hoarseness is another common symptom in primary care, particularly in smokers, but it is actually rare in lung cancer. Laryngoscopy is generally recommended in hoarse patients (see Chapter 17), primarily to identify laryngeal problems.

Finger Clubbing and Lymphadenopathy

Both these features are associated with lung cancer in secondary care but there is little evidence on their diagnostic value in primary care. Referral for a chest X-ray is sensible.

History and Examination

Boxes 7.2 and 7.3 provide aspects of history and examination that should generally be included when there is clinical suspicion of lung cancer. They are by no means exhaustive!

Investigations

As the majority of UK patients with lung cancer present initially with symptoms to primary care, prompt investigation of symptomatic patients is important. The main investigation is the chest X-ray.

Box 7.2   History taking in a patient with a symptom that may be lung cancer

- Sociodemographic characteristics
- General health, any recent changes
- Respiratory symptoms:
  - *Cough:* characteristics, frequency
  - *Haemoptysis:* establish severity, and whether bleeding potentially from other source
  - *Shortness of breath:* nature, any recent change
  - *Chest pain:* site, frequency, intensity
- Non-specific symptoms: weight loss, fatigue, general malaise, loss of appetite
- Relevant past medical history such as frequent chest infections, childhood illnesses
- Family history of lung cancer, other lung disease
- Occupational history (looking particularly for asbestos exposure)
- Detailed smoking history including exposure to environmental smoke
- Recent travel to areas of high TB or HIV prevalence

Box 7.3   Examination of a patient with a symptom that may be lung cancer

- General appearance and vital signs
- Chest:
  - *Shape, expansion*
  - *Examination of lung fields, breath sounds, any added sounds*
  - *Cardiovascular examination*
- Lymph nodes
- Ear, nose and throat examination
- Extremities, particularly finger clubbing, discolouration through smoking

Chest X-ray

This is a simple, inexpensive and accessible investigation. It is appropriate in almost all cases before any referral for specialist investigation. However, a negative X-ray does not completely exclude lung cancer and GPs should be guided by their clinical suspicion. Small lesions may be missed, leading to diagnostic delay. The exact false-negative rate in the detection of early lung cancer on the chest X-ray is difficult to estimate but may be up to a quarter. Even so, the use of a chest X-ray as an initial investigation is undisputed.

Sputum Cytology

This should very rarely be performed before specialist referral, as it may delay the diagnostic process. It is now mainly used in secondary care, when the patient is too ill for invasive investigation. Nevertheless, it is a non-invasive, cheap and simple test. A positive test is clearly very important but no reliance can be put on a negative test. Most cancers detected by sputum cytology are squamous cell carcinomas, which usually occur centrally and have the highest rate of exfoliation of malignant cells. Cytology enhanced by molecular genetics and immunohistochemistry may improve the test performance, although this test is unlikely to be available in primary care. In the future, DNA analysis of sputum slides by automated sputum cytology may improve accuracy.

Other Investigations

It is generally recommended that standard laboratory tests such as full blood count, ESR and electrolytes should be performed as part of the diagnostic work-up in patients with suspected lung cancer. These will provide helpful information on the patient's general health and the presence of any co-morbidity.

Delay in Diagnosis

Currently, there is no direct evidence that early diagnosis reduces mortality. Even so, a shift away from the current pattern of advanced presentation, with a concomitant increase in potentially curative treatments such as lung resection, could impact favourably. Early diagnosis has been associated in several studies with better prospects for operability and with a better prognosis. Certainly, there is considerable international variation, with about 10% of UK lung cancer patients receiving surgical treatment compared with 28% in the US.

Relatively little is known about the reasons why patients delay reporting their symptoms. Individuals frequently fail to recognise symptoms that they have experienced over many months prior to their eventual diagnosis as being serious or 'warranting medical attention'. Once diagnosed, patients typically recall having symptoms for many months. Both chest and systemic symptoms are common but are not perceived to be serious at onset and are not acted upon (with the exception of haemoptysis). Symptoms, even when severe, are attributed to more common, everyday causes.

The reasons for attitudes such as these are complex. A 'nihilistic' attitude is sometimes referred to in relation to lung cancer; there is such a strong perception in the community that lung cancer is 'incurable' and that, beyond smoking cessation, there is little that individuals can do to avoid the disease or facilitate timely diagnosis. These attitudes have important implications for general practice and imply an important educational role; patients need to be encouraged not to ignore symptoms of potential significance. The belief that all lung cancer is incurable and that there is no point in seeking medical help also needs to be challenged.

Further Reading/Key References

Corner J, Hopkinson J, Fitzsimmons D et al 2005 Is late diagnosis of lung cancer inevitable? Interview study of patients' recollections of symptoms before diagnosis. Thorax 60: 314–319

Corner J, Hopkinson J, Roffe L 2005 Experience of health changes and reasons for delay in seeking care: a UK study of the months prior to the diagnosis of lung cancer. Social Science and Medicine 14:1381–1391

Hackshaw A K, Law M R, Wald N J 1997 The accumulated evidence on lung cancer and environmental tobacco smoke. British Medical Journal 15:980–988

Hamilton W, Sharp D 2004 Diagnosis of lung cancer in primary care: a structured review. Family Practice 21:605–611

Hamilton W, Peters T J, Round A et al 2005 What are the clinical features of lung cancer before the diagnosis is made? A population based case-control study. Thorax 60:1059–1065

Koyi H, Hillerdal G, Branden E 2002 Patients' and doctors' delays in the diagnosis of chest tumours. Lung Cancer 35: 53–57

Matakidou A, Eisen T, Houlston R S 2005 Systematic review of the relationship between family history and lung cancer risk. British Journal of Cancer 93:825–833

Scottish Executive 2002 Scottish referral guidelines for suspected cancer. Scottish Executive, London. Available online at: www.scotland.gov.uk/Publications/2002/05/14862/5419

Chapter 8

Urological Cancer

William Hamilton and Tim J. Peters

Epidemiology

Three main cancers arise in the urinary organs: prostate, bladder and kidney. In total they account for nearly one new cancer in every six. Prostate cancer is the commonest of the three, with over 27,000 new cases in the UK annually, followed by bladder with 11,000 and kidney with 6000 new diagnoses. A full-time GP would expect to have at least one new urological cancer diagnosed in their list of patients each year.

Prostate Cancer

Approximately one man in 14 is diagnosed with prostate cancer during his lifetime. However, post-mortem studies show that by 50 years of age, half of men have the histological changes of this cancer and three-quarters have them by the age of 85. The incidence in the UK rose steeply from 1970 to 1995 but has decreased slightly since then. The first phase of the increase was mainly due to the discovery of clinically unsuspected cancers at routine prostatectomy. A second increase occurred in the 1990s as prostate specific antigen (PSA) testing was introduced as an investigative procedure in response to urological symptoms and in some places as a method of screening. The age distribution of new diagnoses is shown in Figure 8.1.

Bladder Cancer

This cancer is much more common in men than women, with a male:female ratio of approximately 2.5:1. The main risk factor is smoking (many metabolites derived from tobacco are excreted through the urine) so the epidemiology mirrors that of lung cancer. The incidence rose steadily

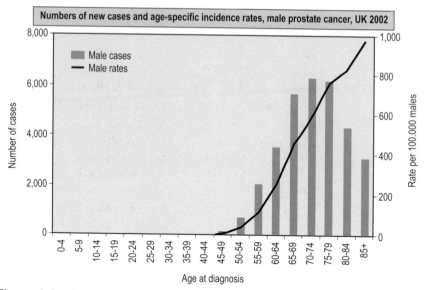

Figure 8.1   Annual incidence of prostate cancer by age group (reproduced with permission from Cancer Research UK, Jan 2006. http://info.cancerresearchuk.org/cancerstats/types/prostate/incidence/)

until 1990 but has fallen since then, with the fall much more marked in men. The risk increases steadily with age.

Kidney Cancer

Again, this is more common in men than women, with a sex ratio of 2:1. It is also largely a disease of older people and, like bladder cancer, the risk increases continuously with increasing age. Unlike bladder cancer, kidney cancer is becoming more common and has nearly doubled in incidence in both sexes over the last 35 years.

Risk Factors

Family history of urological cancer

There is an inherited component to these cancers. A man who has a first-degree relative with prostate cancer has 2–3 times the normal risk of prostate cancer. Furthermore, there are some very rare familial syndromes which incorporate urological cancer, particularly of the kidney or prostate.

In some of these syndromes an aberrant gene has been identified but for the vast majority of men with a positive family history, genetic testing has nothing to offer in quantifying their risk of urological cancer.

Urological Cancer Presentation

There are relatively few ways in which urological cancer can present. Furthermore, urinary symptoms, such as haematuria, may be caused by any of the three cancers in this chapter. To avoid repetition, all such symptoms have been described together, with differences between the three cancers highlighted. This also makes clinical sense as, for example, the investigation of haematuria is aimed at identifying any urological cancer, not just one of them. Of course, such investigation will also include testing for non-malignant conditions such as urinary infection or glomerulonephritis.

Asymptomatic Presentation

This is largely a feature of prostate cancer, with these cancers increasingly detected by PSA testing (see Chapter 2). In the US, over three-quarters of cancers follow this diagnostic pathway; in Europe approximately a quarter do and this proportion is increasing. The UK has one of the lowest rates of PSA screening, though it is increasing in popularity. In our recent UK study of prostate cancers diagnosed between 1998 and 2003, only 8% had been identified following screening of asymptomatic men.

A small proportion of other urological cancers are identified when haematuria is noted on a dipstick performed for other purposes. Around 15% of the population over the age of 40 have urinalysis each year (usually for monitoring of diabetes or hypertension). The proportion of cancers identified by this route is unknown but it is important to act upon an unexpected positive test for haematuria.

The Relationship with Benign Prostatic Hyperplasia

Three-quarters of prostate cancers in the UK are diagnosed following presentation with lower urinary tract symptoms, such as urinary frequency, hesitancy and a poor urinary stream. The term 'prostatism' for this group of symptoms has been replaced by the wider term 'lower urinary tract symptoms', or LUTS, reflecting the fact that not all urinary symptoms in older men are caused by benign prostatic hyperplasia (BPH). BPH is common and so is prostate cancer. Therefore they are often found together, even though studies of the association between BPH and cancer suggest that there is little or no true connection between them.

Even though BPH does not make prostate cancer more likely, it does increase the chance of an incidental cancer being uncovered. It may be discovered as an unexpected finding after prostatectomy for BPH (although the proportion of cancers uncovered in this way has decreased markedly with near universal PSA testing in urology clinics). Now that the standard management of a man with LUTS in primary care includes a PSA test as well as rectal examination, some prostate cancers are found even though these cancers were not the cause of the symptoms.

Symptomatic Presentation

The UK guidelines for urological cancer are drawn together in Box 8.1.

There are six main features of urological cancer. Their frequency is shown in Table 8.1, along with an estimate of the risk of cancer posed by each symptom – that is, the PPV of the single symptoms. All the risks rise with age and are 2–4 times higher in men over the age of 70.

Urinary Retention

Although this can occur with urinary infection, it is most commonly seen in men with enlargement of the prostate. To a large extent, the approximate

---

Box 8.1   Summarised UK guidelines for urgent referral of possible urological cancer

- The following unexplained symptoms may be caused by prostate cancer: erectile dysfunction, haematuria, low back pain, bone pain, weight loss. These patients should have a digital rectal examination (DRE) and a PSA test
- Patients with a hard, irregular prostate
- Patients with an above normal or rising PSA (irrespective of symptoms)
- Patients of any age with painless macroscopic haematuria (after treatment of any urinary infection)
- Patients over 40, with recurrent haematuria and urinary infection
- Patients over 50, with unexplained microscopic haematuria
- Patients of any age with an abdominal mass arising from the urinary tract

Table 8.1 The top six features of urological cancer in primary care

Symptom	Percentage of cancer patients with this symptom			Percentage risk of urological cancer for a patient over 40 reporting this symptom to their GP			
	Prostate	Bladder	Kidney	Prostate	Bladder	Kidney	Total
Acute retention	15	Very rare	Very rare	3	Unknown, probably small	Unknown, probably small	~3
LUTS	>60	Un known, probably small		2–3	Unknown, probably small	Unknown, probably small	2–3
Frank haematuria	15	80 (M) 70 (F)		1	8	1–2	10
Impotence	30	Unknown, probably small		3		Unknown, probably small	3
Weight loss	Mainly with disseminated disease			1		Unknown, probably small	~1
Urinary tract infection	10	70		<1	<1	<<1	~1

3% risk of cancer is not an issue for the GP. This is because the usual management of retention is referral to hospital for catheterisation. While the patient is in hospital the cause of the prostatic enlargement is generally identified. Indeed, prostatectomy is now often performed during or shortly after the admission with retention, so any cancer of the prostate is likely to be identified. This cancer may have been the cause of the prostatic enlargement or may have been a small focus of malignancy within an otherwise benignly enlarged gland.

Lower Urinary Tract Symptoms

This is largely an issue for prostate cancer. In an ideal world, one of these symptoms would stand out as a reasonable discriminator for malignant enlargement of the prostate. However, none does, as shown in Figure 8.2.

Quite simply, a man has a risk of prostate cancer of about 3% if he presents with one of the lower urinary tract symptoms. This risk is not greatly altered by the presence of the other symptoms. Box 8.2 indicates the appropriate investigations for men presenting to primary care with LUTS.

	Positive predictive values for prostate cancer for LUTS, and for pairs of LUTS in combination		
Nocturia	Hesitancy	Frequency/ urgency	
2.2	3.0	2.2	PPV as a single symptom
3.3	2.8	3.2	Nocturia
	2.0	4.7	Hesitancy
		3.1	Frequency/ urgency

Figure 8.2 Positive predictive values for prostate cancer for LUTS and for pairs of LUTS in combination (adapted from Hamilton et al 2006, by permission of the British Journal of General Practice).

Box 8.2   Investigation of a patient with LUTS

- Perform a rectal examination
- Discuss a PSA

Rectal Examination

This is the main (perhaps only) examination that is of any use in identifying prostate cancer. The normal prostate is similar in consistency to a contracted calf muscle. The whole posterior surface should be easily palpable and both lobes identifiable separately. A malignant prostate may be palpable as a nodule, as an asymmetry in the two lobes, as a loss of the median sulcus or (most commonly) as an increased hardness of the gland, variously described as woody, stony or craggy. If one of these features is present, the risk of cancer is about 12%. This compares with a risk of 2.8% when the gland feels benignly enlarged. Of course, this risk of 2.8% is roughly the risk that the patient had from his symptoms. In this respect, a benign-feeling prostate is not that reassuring. Some cancers may be too deep within the gland to be palpable.

Discuss a PSA

The only test that is of value in the primary care diagnosis of prostate cancer is a PSA. In this situation, the PSA test is being used as an investigation, not as a screening tool in a (generally) asymptomatic population of men. The distinction is important and sometimes not fully appreciated. When a patient attends with LUTS he is asking for diagnosis and treatment of a symptom. The treatment of the symptom is different for the two main diagnoses, BPH and cancer. BPH may well be treated medically unless symptoms are severe, bothersome and persistent; cancer will often be treated surgically. The argument used by opponents of PSA testing in men with LUTS is that some cancers will be identified that were not the cause of the man's symptoms. This is so but it is likely that surgical management will be chosen or at least strongly considered, as it will treat the two conditions present, BPH and cancer, simultaneously. Therefore, a PSA test may well be appropriate when a man has LUTS, as it will guide management. However, this should be discussed with the man and fully informed consent is crucial.* Indeed, it is

---

*We know that this sounds like the answer to an MRCGP viva (and so by definition suspect). However, the consequences of testing without discussion may be bad – for the doctor as well as the patient. As we write, a clinician is being sued for diagnosing prostate cancer when he hadn't told the man he was being tested.

possible that his reasons for consulting the GP included a desire to find out if he had cancer or not, not just for treatment of his symptoms.

The usual threshold quoted for a PSA test is 4.0 ng/ml, although patients below this figure may have cancer and patients above it may not. If the PSA is above 4.0 ng/ml, the risk of prostate cancer is around 24–38%. Referral to a specialist clinic is then clearly required, with clear and comprehensive information about the investigative and treatment options continuing to be important, especially given the lack of a definitive evidence base for the latter.

Haematuria

This is a key symptom for bladder and for kidney cancer and it may also appear with prostate cancer. As Table 8.1 showed, the overall risk of a cancer for a person over the age of 40 with frank haematuria is nearly 10%. It is much lower in those with microscopic haematuria identified as part of a screening examination of the urine. The precise risk of cancer with microscopic haematuria is hotly debated. In all studies of patients with microscopic haematuria identified at screening, only a small proportion of patients with a positive test were fully investigated, leaving some doubt about whether cancer could have been present in those who had not been investigated. Two studies of men over 50 and 60 years of age with screen-detected haematuria calculated PPVs of 4.7% and 5.3% respectively for urological cancer. Two-thirds of these cancers were bladder tumours and the remainder prostate tumours. In contrast, a study of 100 men under 40 years of age found no cancers.

What is the Nature of the Bleeding?

The idea behind this question is that blood at the end of the stream (terminal haematuria) is more likely to originate from the bladder or the prostate. Blood throughout the stream can come from anywhere in the urinary tract.

Box 8.3   Questions in a patient with frank haematuria

- What is the nature of the bleeding? Is the blood present throughout the urine or predominantly at the end or beginning of the stream?
- What other symptoms are present?

> **Box 8.4   Examination and investigations in a patient with haematuria and no other symptoms**
>
> - Measure the blood pressure
> - Urinalysis for protein
> - MSU to confirm and quantify the haematuria and identify infection

What Other Symptoms are Present?

This is essentially a search for other causes of haematuria. Renal colic suggests stones or the loin pain-haematuria syndrome. Symptoms of urinary infection should allow this diagnosis to be made confidently (though urinary infection may be an initial manifestation of cancer). Progressive fatigue may suggest advancing glomerulonephritis and the haematuria will usually be accompanied by proteinuria.

The first two of these items are targeted at identifying glomerulonephritis. The MSU is the only test of appreciable value when cancer is being considered. Although urine cytology is available and has a sensitivity of over 80% for bladder cancer, its general performance statistics, including the specificity and in particular the NPV, are such that a negative test would not allow the GP to be confident in stopping investigation. The MSU has two functions. First, it will confirm that bleeding is present; urinalysis sticks are extremely sensitive, though, and may be positive even when there is insignificant haematuria. Second, it may identify a urine infection.

On most occasions, the tests are negative. In these circumstances it is reasonable to repeat the urine testing after a few weeks, especially in a premenopausal woman. If the haematuria is persistent, urological referral for investigation of possible cancer is wise, though the likeliest outcome is that no cause for the bleeding will be found.

Urinary Tract Infections

Bladder cancer can present as recurrent urinary infections. Indeed, the association between the two conditions is strong enough that it has been suggested that recurrent infections may be part of the causal pathway, particularly for squamous cell bladder cancer. Bladder cancer is a late manifestation of infection with schistosomiasis but in this infection the eggs of the parasite become buried in the tissue of the bladder wall, provoking inflammation. For bacterial urinary infections, the link with bladder cancer is much more likely to be that cancer predisposes to urinary infection, rather than vice versa.

For the GP, this probably does not matter. In patients with recurrent or persistent infection, an MSU will be taken (indeed, probably several will be taken). As long as attention is given to ensuring that any haematuria is noted, it is unlikely that cancer will be missed. If there is haematuria present (and there usually will be) it is important to repeat the test after the infection has been treated. Persistent haematuria requires investigation.

Impotence

One recent study has identified an association between impotence and a future diagnosis of prostate cancer. The risk was calculated at 3% and the impotence was reported often many months before the cancer was diagnosed. Routine management of impotence in primary care does not usually include a rectal examination or a PSA test. These are worth considering.

Further Reading/Key References

Bruyninckx R, Buntinx F, Aertgeerts B, Van Casteren V 2003 The diagnostic value of macroscopic haematuria for the diagnosis of urological cancer in general practice. British Journal of General Practice 53:31–35

Del Mar D 2000 Evidence based case report: Asymptomatic haematuria . . . in the doctor. British Medical Journal 320:165–166

Hamilton W, Sharp D 2004 Symptomatic diagnosis of prostate cancer in primary care: a structured review. British Journal of General Practice 54:617–621

Hamilton W, Sharp D, Peters T, Round A 2006 Clinical features of prostate cancer before diagnosis: a population-based case-control study. British Journal of General Practice 56:756–762

Kjaer S K, Knudsen J B, Sorensen B L, Moller Jensen O 1989 The Copenhagen case-control study of bladder cancer. V. Review of the role of urinary-tract infection. Acta Oncologica 28:631–636

Moore L E, Wilson R T, Campleman S L 2005 Lifestyle factors, exposures, genetic susceptibility and renal cell cancer risk: a review. Cancer Investigation 23:240–255

Chapter 9

Skin Cancers
Richard D. Neal

Epidemiology

Primary skin cancers are extremely common, with an estimated 100,000 new cases diagnosed each year in the UK. They are also important, as early detection and treatment result in excellent survival; conversely, survival rates are poor for advanced disease. Skin cancers are becoming more common and public awareness of suspicious skin lesions is increasing. This has led to more skin lesions being presented to GPs for assessment. Most skin cancers are preventable; about four out of five malignant melanomas in the UK are caused by exposure to the sun. Throughout this chapter the three primary skin cancers will be discussed separately but where there are aspects in common, these will be highlighted.

Malignant Melanoma

This is the most important of the primary skin cancers in that it causes an estimated 1700 deaths from 7300 cases per annum in the UK. This equates to roughly one new case every 5 years per full-time GP. It has been estimated that one in every 95 white people will develop a melanoma during their lifetime. It accounts for 2% of all cancers and 1% of all cancer deaths. The increase in incidence by age is illustrated in Figure 9.1.

The incidence in the UK is one of the highest in Europe but is considerably lower than in Australia, New Zealand and the white population of America. The incidence has tripled over the past 25 years and continues to increase. This is due to a combination of factors, including diagnosis of earlier lesions and increasing sun exposure.

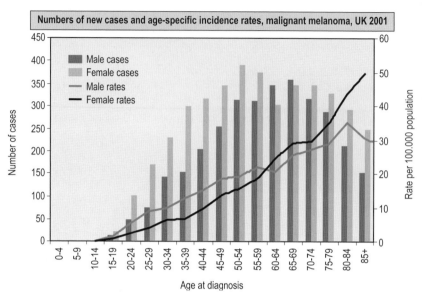

Figure 9.1   Number of new cases of malignant melanoma and age-specific annual incidence, UK 2001 (reproduced with permission from Cancer Research UK, Jan 2006 http://info.cancerresearchuk.org/cancerstats/types/melanoma/incidence/).

Risk Factors

Melanomas develop as a result of a complex interaction between environmental and genetic factors. Perhaps the most important determinant of developing melanoma is skin damage from ultraviolet light. As a consequence, melanoma is 80% more common in whites compared to non-whites and in white people with fairer skin. About four out of five malignant melanomas in the UK are caused by sun exposure. A positive family history is present in 5–10% of patients and increases risk 2–8-fold.

People with dysplastic naevus syndrome are also at increased risk. Dysplastic naevi are melanocytic lesions that can be precursors of melanoma. These lesions are identified by certain clinical and histological features: they are larger than most naevi; their borders are fuzzy and irregular; pigmentation is varied and irregular; and they are most commonly seen on areas exposed to the sun. The presence of dysplastic naevi, along with a positive family history, results in a markedly increased risk.

Basal Cell Carcinoma

Also known as 'rodent ulcer', basal cell carcinoma accounts for 40,000 new diagnoses per year in the UK. Most GPs will see a basal carcinoma annually. The peak incidence is in patients aged 60–80 years. They develop in the deep basal cell layer of the epidermis and are commonest on the face and neck, typically around the nose, ear, cheek and temple. Whilst far more common than malignant melanoma, they very rarely metastasise and so cause far less morbidity and mortality. However, treatment is needed to prevent deeper ulceration and local spread. There is a tendency for these lesions to recur (5% at 5 years), hence patients need to be vigilant once an initial lesion has been treated.

Squamous Cell Carcinoma

This accounts for 10,000 new diagnoses per year in the UK, with 400 deaths annually, so a GP would expect to see a new case every 3–4 years. They are commoner in men, patients over 55 years of age and Caucasians living closer to the equator. Like the other primary skin cancers, they are found in parts of the body exposed to sunlight. Although more aggressive than basal cell carcinomas, with the potential for spread to local lymph nodes, squamous cell carcinoma causes less morbidity and mortality than malignant melanoma. Treatment is needed to prevent deeper ulceration and local spread.

Risk Factors for Basal Cell and Squamous Cell Carcinoma

The risk factors for these two primary skin cancers are similar. The risk is greater for both with increasing sun exposure, especially sunburn; like melanoma, around 90% of cases are believed to be attributable to increased exposure to the sun. Both are more common in people with fair skin, light hair and light eyes. Both are more likely in immuno-suppressed patients (for example, those with organ transplants) and in patients with scarring (particularly wounds that have been slow to heal) or traumatised skin (especially after irradiation). Xeroderma pigmentosum is a rare autosomal dominant form of non-melanoma skin cancer in patients under 40 years of age, due to a defective DNA repair mechanism. Past treatment with arsenicals (previously found in various tonics) carries a small risk of squamous cell carcinoma. Precursor lesions are actinic (solar) keratoses and Bowen's disease (squamous cell carcinoma in situ). Smoking pipes and cigars (lip lesions), industrial carcinogens (tars, oils) and infection with the human papilloma virus also predispose to squamous cell carcinoma.

> **Box 9.1   UK guidelines (2005 version) recommendations for urgent referral of possible skin cancer**
>
> - If a melanoma is suspected then an urgent referral to a dermatologist or other suitable specialist with experience of melanoma diagnosis should be made and excision in primary care avoided
> - All persistent or slowly evolving or unresponsive skin lesions should be referred
> - All lesions excised should be sent to the pathology laboratory
> - A pathological report should always be sent with the referral
> - All pigmented lesions that are not viewed as suspicious of melanoma but are excised should have a lateral excision margin of 2 mm of clinically normal skin and cut to include subcutaneous fat in depth
> - For lesions with a low level of clinical suspicion, change should be determined over time by the use of photographs and a marker scale or ruler

Skin Cancer Presentation

Primary skin cancers can be difficult to diagnose, especially early lesions. The golden rule is to refer for specialist opinion and biopsy if there is any doubt. The UK guidelines for referral are summarised in Box 9.1.

The quality of evidence underpinning referral guidance is poor. This is because of a lack of research regarding the clinical epidemiology of symptoms and clusters of symptoms, indicative of possible skin cancer. Hence the guidance is based upon the best evidence to date and this is predominantly reliant on the research findings from patients referred for assessment rather than those who consult in primary care.

Malignant Melanoma

The majority of these are reported to primary care. Many are first identified by relatives rather than by the patients themselves. One of the difficulties facing GPs is that people develop new (benign) moles throughout their life. Furthermore, some of these continue to grow, again benignly. We are all born with no moles and die with around a hundred. This, combined with an increased awareness of skin cancer, has led to more patients presenting more moles for assessment to doctors.

Change in an existing pigmented skin lesion is the most common presentation. This usually takes place over the course of weeks or months.

If the timespan is days rather than weeks, then the lesion is more likely to be inflammatory than malignant. Most commonly, the lesion changes in two dimensions at least, so it becomes wider but also rises above the surrounding skin. Other symptoms include itching and asymmetry. Later signs are ulceration, bleeding and tenderness.

Overall, the trunk is the commonest location in men and the limbs in women. More rarely, they can occur in mucous membranes such as the digestive tract and the vagina. Well-reported but rare locations are the eye and the sole of the foot. The commonest initial site for spread is the regional lymph nodes, followed by skin and subcutaneous tissue. Metastatic spread most commonly occurs to the lungs, liver, brain and bone. The first presentation may be with metastases.

Typical melanomas are shown in Figures 9.2 and 9.3.

Basal Cell Carcinoma

These are most commonly found on the face, often associated with sun damage and are very rare in non-hair bearing skin (Figs 9.4 and 9.5). They are usually very slow growing and noticeable growth over a period of less than 2 months is unusual. Multiple lesions may occur. Typically, they present as a nodular or nodular ulcerative lesion that is unsightly but otherwise asymptomatic; this often resembles a papule elevated above the surrounding skin, with a pearly appearance and overlapping telangiectasia. However, they can present in other ways, including flatter lesions,

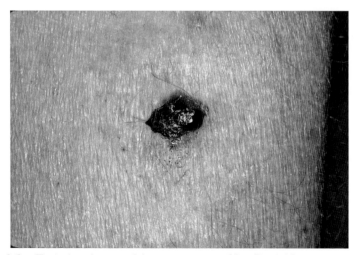

Figure 9.2 Typical melanoma (photo courtesy of Ian Daniels).

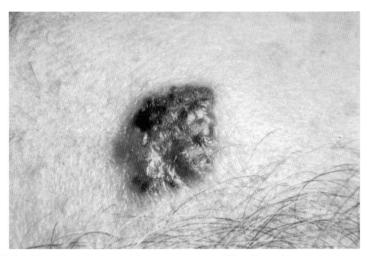

Figure 9.3   Typical melanoma (photo courtesy of Ian Daniels).

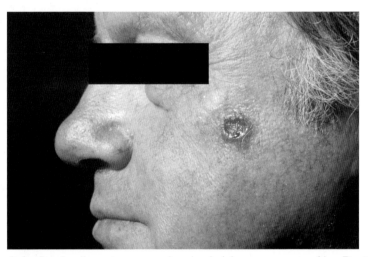

Figure 9.4   Basal cell carcinoma on the cheek (photo courtesy of Ian Daniels).

non-healing erosive ulcers or pigmented papules. If suspected, a non-urgent referral should be made.

Squamous Cell Carcinoma

These are classically nodular, sometimes with central ulceration or ulcerated with a raised everted nodular edge. If the hyperkeratotic scale is

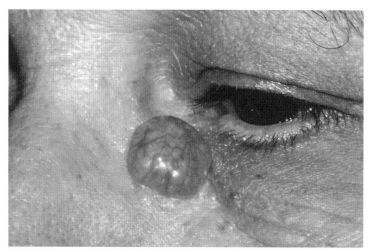

Figure 9.5   Basal cell carcinoma (photo courtesy of Ian Daniels).

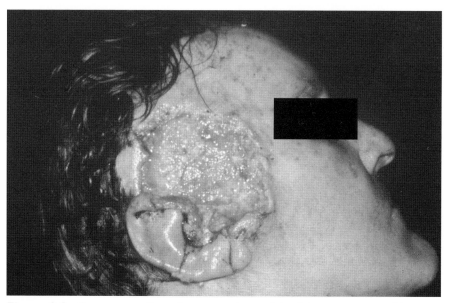

Figure 9.6   Squamous cell carcinoma on the earlobe (photo courtesy of Ian Daniels).

removed, the tumour bleeds. They usually occur on exposed parts of the skin (Fig. 9.6). The risk of a non-healing skin lesion in primary care being a squamous cell carcinoma is 2–4%. An in situ lesion, or Bowen's disease, is usually a single, red, well-demarcated and thin plaque ranging in diameter from a few millimetres to several centimetres. Between 3% and 5% will develop into squamous cell carcinomas with a high potential for metastasis. Non-healing (often keratanising or crusted) lesions greater than 1 cm with significant induration on palpation, with expansion over 8 weeks may be squamous cell carcinomas and an urgent referral should be made. These lesions are particularly common on the face, scalp and back of the hand.

Treatment

Primary care excision of suspicious lesions

Lesions that are removed in general practice (whether by design or 'accident') do not have a worse survival outcome than secondary care excisions. Even so, if the lesion is thought to be malignant, referral is wise and indeed is encouraged by the referral guidelines. The problem is that it is very difficult for a GP to be sure that there is a negligible risk of malignancy. In these 'low-risk' excision biopsies, the rules in the guidelines are very sensible: ensure a 2 mm margin is taken around the lesion and some subcutaneous fat is included (this allows accurate assessment of the malignancy if it surprisingly turns out to be one). Crucially, every skin lesion must be sent for histology; omitting this is a classic medicolegal blunder.

Malignant Melanoma

All suspicious lesions should have an excision biopsy with margins of 2 mm all around the lesion. If the lesion is confirmed to be a malignant melanoma, then a wide local excision with margins dictated by the Breslow thickness is recommended (1 cm margin if Breslow <1 mm, 1–2 cm if 1–2 mm, 1–2 cm (but 2 cm preferred) if 2.1–4 mm and 2–3 cm for >4 mm). If nodes are involved at diagnosis then a node clearance is undertaken. For locally invasive or metastatic lesions, radiotherapy or chemotherapy may be recommended.

Basal Cell Carcinoma

Diagnosis is usually confirmed by biopsy. The aim of treatment is local destruction of the tumour, once the diagnosis is established (this is often made clinically in recurrent tumours). The tumour may be removed surgically or by other locally destructive means. These include cryotherapy (especially if there are multiple superficial lesions) and curettage and cautery (especially if the patient is infirm or for lesions on the trunk and arms). Radiotherapy, photodynamic therapy and topical application of chemotherapeutic drugs may also be used. The prognosis is excellent and it is normal practice not to follow up if the tumour has been fully removed.

If the patient has had many basal cell carcinomas then follow-up should be aimed at early detection of further local recurrence.

Squamous Cell Carcinoma

Again, the aim of treatment is local destruction of the tumour and this is usually undertaken surgically, although radiation therapy is sometimes used. A tumour that is located close to an orifice may require more extensive surgery.

Further Reading/Key References

Roberts D, Anstey A V, Barlow R J et al 2002 UK guidelines for the management of cutaneous melanoma. British Journal of Dermatology 146:7–17
Scottish Intercollegiate Guidelines Network (SIGN) 2003 Cutaneous melanoma. Scottish Intercollegiate Guidelines Network, Edinburgh. Available online at: www.sign.ac.uk/guidelines/published/index.html#Cancer

Chapter 10

Ovarian Cancer

Clare Bankhead

Epidemiology

Ovarian cancer is the most common gynaecological cancer in women, with around 6800 new cases diagnosed each year in the UK and 4600 deaths. This equates to roughly one new case every 5 years per full-time GP. It is predominantly a disease of older, postmenopausal women. The incidence rises steeply after the menopause, with more than 80% of cases being diagnosed in women over 50 years (Fig. 10.1).

Until recently the incidence of ovarian cancer in the UK had been steadily increasing by around 1% a year. Much of that increase was observed in women aged over 65 years, with the rates in women under 65 remaining relatively stable. For the last 10 years or so, the overall incidence rate has stabilised. This levelling off may be due to the widespread use of the oral contraceptive pill, which appears to exert a protective influence.

Whilst the 5-year survival associated with early-stage ovarian cancer is very good (around 70%), the majority of cases are diagnosed at an advanced stage of disease, at which point the 5-year survival rate is poor (15%). Correspondingly, the overall 5-year survival rate is low, at around 30–40%, with ovarian cancer the fourth most common cause of cancer death in women, accounting for 6% of all female cancer deaths. The challenge in diagnosing ovarian cancer, therefore, is how it can be identified earlier when there is the potential for an increased survival rate.

Risk Factors

Several putative risk factors have been investigated such as parity, twin pregnancies, breastfeeding, infertility and fertility treatment, oral contraceptives, tubal ligation, hormone replacement therapy, use of talcum powder,

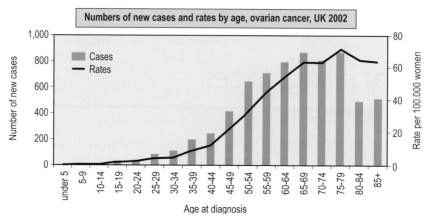

Figure 10.1   Annual incidence of ovarian cancer by age group, 2002 (reproduced with permission from Cancer Research UK, Jan 2006. http://info.cancerresearchuk.org/cancerstats/types/ovary/incidence/?a=5441).

obesity, polycystic ovary syndrome and endometriosis, infective agents, the use of some medications, and molecular biology and genetics. Only age and genetic influences are strongly associated with the disease.

Parity

The risk of ovarian cancer is higher in nulliparous women than in parous women. Compared with women who have had four or more children, the odds ratio of ovarian cancer for nulliparous women is 2.4 and that for women with one pregnancy is 2.1.

Infertility and Fertility Treatment

Infertility appears to carry a risk over and above that of nulliparity. Women who had been attempting pregnancy for more than 5 years had an odds ratio of 2.7 when compared to women who had been trying to conceive for less than a year. The relationship between fertility treatment and ovarian cancer is controversial; the problem in assessing the risk associated with fertility treatment is disentangling the effects of infertility (the cause of treatment) from the treatment itself.

Oral Contraceptives

The use of oral contraceptives is protective, perhaps due to cessation of ovulation or to a reduction in endogenous oestrogen production. The protective effect of the oral contraceptive pill (odds ratio of 0.66 in ever versus never users) appears to be prolonged, with no significant differences between women who cease pill use within the last 10 years compared to those who stopped over 20 years ago.

Tubal Ligation

This has a protective effect, with an estimated risk reduction of between 18% and 70%. The biological mechanism for this association is not well understood. Hysterectomy may also reduce risk.

Hormone Replacement Therapy

Whether hormone replacement therapy (HRT) plays a role in ovarian cancer risk remains uncertain but if it does, then any such effect appears to be small.

Genetic Predisposition

Mutations in the breast cancer genes BRCA1 and BRCA2 and hereditary non-polyposis colorectal cancer (HNPCC) genes are associated with an increased risk of ovarian cancer, although only about 10% of ovarian carcinomas occur in women known to have these mutations (see Chapters 3 and 5). In women with a BRCA1 mutation, the lifetime risk of developing ovarian cancer is approximately 1 in 2, compared with an approximate 1 in 48 risk for women without the mutation. By the age of 70, 39% of BRCA1 mutation carriers and 11% of BRCA2 carriers will have developed ovarian cancer. In women carrying a HNPCC mutation, the lifetime risk of ovarian cancer is about 12%. Women who have inherited a gene mutation that puts them at high risk of ovarian cancer may consider having prophylactic surgery or regular screening for ovarian cancer although such screening is only currently available as part of a research study.

Prophylactic Surgery

Prophylactic oophorectomy decreases the risk of BRCA mutation-related gynaecological cancers in BRCA1 and BRCA2 mutation carriers. Prophylactic surgery is usually performed before the age of 40 years, as the incidence in these women starts to increase after this age. Of great importance is that these women have access to the appropriate specialists, as such a procedure can have extensive psychological consequences.

Delay in Presentation and Diagnosis of Ovarian Cancer

Most ovarian cancers are diagnosed at an advanced stage. This has been blamed upon the insidious nature of the disease and the vagueness of the symptoms. Specifically, the symptoms may be interpreted by women as being normal changes in the body, such as the effects of childbearing, menopause and ageing.

As with several other cancers, the relationship between the duration of symptoms and the outcome is complex. Studies of the effect of delay on clinical outcomes have produced contradictory results, with some research demonstrating that longer patient delay is associated with more advanced disease and total (patient and system) delays leading to poorer survival, whilst others have shown that reduced system delay is associated with poor prognosis. This latter observation may indicate that health professionals recognise symptoms associated with advanced-stage or aggressive disease relatively easily and refer these women promptly to specialist care, but that such management has little effect on survival for women with an already poor prognosis.

Many women with ovarian cancer consider that their diagnosis had been delayed. Perhaps the most important explanation was that neither the woman nor the doctors associated her symptoms with possible malignancy.

Ovarian Cancer Presentation

Asymptomatic 'presentation'

The popular image of ovarian cancer is of the 'silent killer'. The percentage of women who are diagnosed in the absence of symptoms ranges between 5% and 26%, depending on whether symptom information was collected directly from women or from medical records.

Symptomatic Presentation

A variety of symptoms are observed in women with ovarian cancer and these may be present for over a year before the diagnosis is made. Much of the research into symptoms associated with ovarian cancer has been retrospective or has used hospital medical records, which may introduce marked biases into the results. Furthermore, the studies have rarely been based in primary care, so the risk of ovarian cancer from individual symptoms in that setting is largely unknown. The studies have also been relatively small and at times had conflicting results.

In approximate order of frequency, the symptoms most commonly reported are as follows:

- abdominal or back pain
- abdominal bloating/abdominal distension. Abdominal distension and abdominal bloating are used in this chapter with different meanings: *distension* means continuous swelling, often increasing over time; *bloating* is used to mean intermittent swelling. Women may use these terms interchangeably (generally preferring bloating) and often the two concepts are merged in research papers. It is likely that abdominal distension, rather than bloating, is indicative of ovarian cancer, despite the choice of the word 'bloating' in the referral guidelines shown in Box 10.1
- urinary symptoms
- fatigue
- bowel irregularities
- loss of appetite and loss of weight.

Symptoms in Early- and Advanced-Stage Disease

Local symptoms, such as urinary or pelvic symptoms, predominate in early-stage disease. In advanced-stage disease, gastrointestinal symptoms, fatigue, abdominal distension, bowel irregularities and weight change may also be experienced. Such symptoms are also more common in women with invasive, as opposed to borderline, tumours. Respiratory symptoms may arise with severe ascites or when there are lung metastases.

Box 10.1   UK guidelines (2005 version) recommendations for urgent referral of possible ovarian cancer

- Refer urgently for ultrasound women with a palpable abdominal or pelvic mass that is not obviously fibroids, gastrointestinal or urinary. If the scan is suggestive of cancer (or unavailable), an urgent referral should be made
- In patients with vague, non-specific, unexplained abdominal symptoms such as bloating, constipation, abdominal pain, back pain or urinary symptoms, abdominal palpation should be done and pelvic examination considered

Comparative Data Between Cases and Controls

Five case–control studies have compared the symptoms experienced by women diagnosed with ovarian cancer to a control group. Elevated odds ratios (but with a large variation between studies) were observed for pelvic/abdominal/back pain and abdominal bloating in four studies, abdominal swelling or enlargement and urinary problems in three studies, and loss of appetite and fatigue in two studies. Many other symptoms were found to be significant in only one of the five studies.

In one study, the PPV of abdominal pain presented to primary care in a woman over 30 years was estimated to be 0.34%. This symptom was chosen as it was the most common in cases. This very low PPV illustrates the difficulty GPs have in diagnosing ovarian cancer when a woman has a single symptom.

Symptom Complexes or Combinations

It is slightly easier when a woman has several symptoms. Two studies examined this. One looked at clusters of three symptoms and produced a set of 10 different combinations, which included three of the following: bloating or fullness, distended or hard abdomen, pelvic or abdominal discomfort, fatigue, gas/nausea/indigestion and weight change. Each of these 10 combinations was reported by 26–39% of cases, compared with 2% or less of controls. In the other study, 43% of ovarian cancer cases experienced bloating, increased abdominal size and urinary urgency compared with 8% of the clinic controls, giving an odds ratio of 9.4. Therefore, when a woman has one of the symptoms of ovarian cancer, her GP should ask about the other symptoms and examine the abdomen. With multiple symptoms, a pelvic examination is warranted.

Implications for Primary Care

Referral decisions are difficult for GPs, due to the relative rarity of the condition, the vagueness of symptoms and the fact that potential symptoms commonly occur in other conditions. An indication of this referral dilemma is that, currently, around 40% of women diagnosed with ovarian cancer are initially referred to clinics other than gynae-oncology. If a GP suspects the presence of ovarian cancer, an urgent referral should be made to a dedicated diagnostic centre at the nearest cancer unit. Surgery should be undertaken by a subspecialty trained gynaecological oncology surgeon, since this improves survival.

Further Reading/Key References

Bankhead C, Kehoe S, Austoker J 2005 Symptoms associated with diagnosis of ovarian cancer: a systematic review. BJOG: International Journal of Obstetrics and Gynaecology 112:857–865

Ferrell B, Smith S, Cullinane C, Melancon C 2003 Symptom concerns of women with ovarian cancer. Journal of Pain and Symptom Management 25:528–538

Friedman G, Skilling J, Udaltsova N, Smith L 2005 Early symptoms of ovarian cancer: a case–control study without recall bias. Family Practice 22:548–553

Goff B, Mandel L, Melancon C, Muntz H 2004 Frequency of symptoms of ovarian cancer in women presenting to primary care clinics. Journal of the American Medical Association 291:2705–2712

Latifeh I, Marsden D, Robertson G, Gebski V, Hacker N 2005 Presenting symptoms of epithelial ovarian cancer. Australian and New Zealand Journal of Obstetrics and Gynaecology 45:211–214

Olson S, Mignone L, Nakraseive C et al 2001 Symptoms of ovarian cancer. Obstetrics and Gynecology 98:212–217

Paulsen T, Kaern J, Kjaerheim K et al 2005 Symptoms and referral of women with epithelial ovarian tumors. International Journal of Gynecology and Obstetrics 88:31–37

Smith L, Morris C, Yasmeen S et al 2005 Ovarian cancer: can we make the clinical diagnosis earlier? Cancer 104:1398

Vine M, Calingaert B, Berchuck A, Schildkraut J 2003 Characterization of prediagnostic symptoms among primary epithelial ovarian cancer cases and controls. Gynecological Oncology 90:75–82

Chapter 11

Upper Gastrointestinal Cancers

Una Macleod and Elizabeth Mitchell

Epidemiology

Over 23,000 cases of upper gastrointestinal cancers are diagnosed in the UK each year with more than 20,000 deaths; this accounts for 13% of all cancer deaths. It is estimated that upper gastrointestinal cancer is the cause of 1.3 million deaths worldwide each year.

Oesophageal Cancer

Oesophageal cancer is the ninth most common UK cancer, with about 7500 new cases each year. It is more common in older people (Fig. 11.1) and has been increasing in incidence over the last few decades.

Stomach Cancer

Stomach cancer is the fourth most common malignancy and the second most frequent cause of cancer-related death in the world. It is also more common in older people (Fig. 11.2) but has been declining in incidence over the last five decades.

Patients at Higher Risk

Between 75% and 90% of cancers arising in the oesophagus are related to tobacco smoking and/or alcohol consumption. Long-standing gastro-oesophageal reflux disease (GORD), obesity and being male are other risk factors for oesophageal cancer. Stomach cancer may also be causally

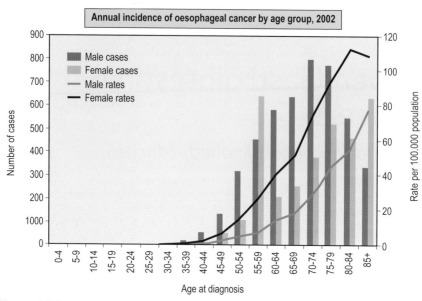

Figure 11.1   Annual incidence of oesophageal cancer by age group, 2002 (reproduced with permission from Cancer Research UK, Jan 2006. http://info.cancerresearchuk.org/cancerstats/types/oesophagus/incidence/).

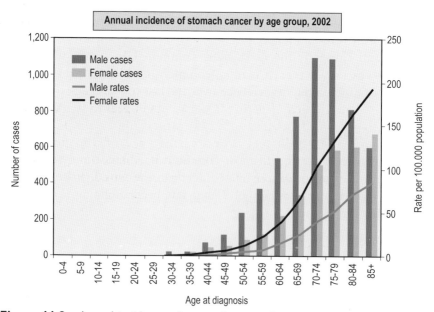

Figure 11.2   Annual incidence of stomach cancer by age group, 2002 (reproduced with permission from Cancer Research UK, Jan 2006. http://info.cancerresearchuk.org/cancerstats/types/stomach/incidence/).

related to tobacco, although this is more contentious. A number of disorders have been associated with increased risk of stomach cancer, including chronic atrophic gastritis, gastric polyps, gastric ulcer, cholecystitis, pernicious anaemia and (in some parts of the world) schistosomiasis. There is convincing evidence that diets high in fruit and vegetables are associated with a reduced incidence of stomach cancer and weaker evidence for a reduction in oesophageal cancer.

Barrett's Oesophagus

Barrett's oesophagus is a premalignant condition characterised by columnar epithelial metaplasia of the distal oesophagus. It may be induced by long-standing GORD and is associated with an 80-fold increased risk of adenocarcinoma of the oesophagus. The risk is greater if there is a long segment (>7 cm) of the oesophagus affected.

Helicobacter pylori

Helicobacter pylori infection is widely present in the population but causes no harm to the majority of people. However, it is associated with both duodenal ulcers and gastric cancer. Distal stomach cancer is strongly associated with life-long infection with *H. pylori*. While peptic ulcer disease may be cured by treatment of *H. pylori*, the potential to reduce the risk of gastric cancer is more contentious.

Antiulcer Drugs

Although debated at great length, there does not appear to be a causal link between H_2-receptor blockers and gastric cancer. Studies examining a link between proton pump inhibitors and gastric cancer have similarly not shown any increased risk, although there is little information on long-term use. However, acid suppression may mask the symptoms of cancer, so even if it does not cause cancer, it may delay its identification.

Symptomatic Presentation

The NICE guidelines are summarised in Boxes 11.1 and 11.2.

In addition to the symptoms listed, an urgent referral should also be made for patients presenting with either unexplained upper abdominal pain and weight loss, with or without back pain, an upper abdominal mass without dyspepsia or obstructive jaundice (an alternative is an urgent ultrasound).

> **Box 11.1   UK Guidelines (2005 version) recommendations for urgent referral for endoscopy**
>
> - Patients of any age with dyspepsia who present with any of the following:
>   - chronic gastrointestinal bleeding
>   - dysphagia
>   - progressive unintentional weight loss
>   - persistent vomiting
>   - iron deficiency anaemia
>   - epigastric mass
>   - suspicious barium meal result
> - Patients aged 55 years and older with unexplained and persistent recent-onset dyspepsia alone

> **Box 11.2   UK guidelines (2005 version) recommendations for urgent referral for further investigation of possible upper gastrointestinal cancer**
>
> Patients with unexplained worsening of their dyspepsia and known to have any of the following risk factors:
> - Barrett's oesophagus
> - dysplasia, atrophic gastritis or intestinal metaplasia
> - peptic ulcer surgery more than 20 years ago
> - unexplained weight loss or iron deficiency anaemia in the absence of dyspepsia
> - persistent vomiting and weight loss in the absence of dyspepsia

Patients aged less than 55 years do not require referral for endoscopy in the absence of 'alarm' symptoms. Patients being referred urgently for endoscopy should ideally be free from acid suppression medication, including proton pump inhibitors or H_2-receptor antagonists, for a minimum of 2 weeks.

Common Symptoms

Oesophageal and stomach cancers present with similar symptoms. Common symptoms in both are dysphagia, weight loss, anaemia and vomiting. Symptoms more commonly seen in oesophageal cancer are heartburn and reflux; in stomach cancer, epigastric pain. Many of these symptoms are extremely common in primary care. As always, GPs need to distinguish those patients whose symptoms may be due to cancer from the much larger number of patients whose symptoms arise from benign, self-limiting illness. Upper GI symptoms (mainly dyspepsia) account for about 5% of a GP's workload. In addition, many patients self-medicate and may never present to primary care. About a third of patients with gastric cancer have a long history of dyspepsia and about 80% report some epigastric pain or dyspepsia.

At an early stage, gastric cancer is symptomless. Over time, patients typically develop vague and non-specific symptoms, for instance mild upper gastrointestinal discomfort or heartburn, flatulence, abdominal fullness prematurely after meals and excessive belching. When the cancer is more extensive then weight loss, anaemia, anorexia, haematemesis and vomiting are frequent.

Dyspepsia

Dyspepsia is defined broadly to include patients with recurrent epigastric pain, heartburn or acid regurgitation, with or without bloating, nausea or vomiting. The most common causes are GORD, peptic ulcer disease and non-ulcer dyspepsia. It occurs in up to 40% of the population and a quarter of these consult their GP. Referral for endoscopy is made in only 1% of sufferers and in these referred patients, cancers are very rare, occurring in 3% of endoscopies.

Although most patients with dyspepsia have a benign cause, patients consulting with dyspepsia often worry that their symptoms are due to a serious illness, most commonly cancer. Dyspepsia on its own is rarely, if ever, due to upper gastrointestinal cancer, especially in patients under 55 years. Its relevance lies in its associated symptoms. Attempts have been made to identify whether symptom subgroups aid diagnosis, although this approach has not as yet proven helpful clinically. Nonetheless, in assessing a patient with dyspepsia it is important to identify associated symptoms.

Box 11.3　Questions in a patient with dyspepsia

- How long has the pain been present and what are the features of this pain?
- Has there been any bleeding?
- Has there been any persistent vomiting?
- Has there been any progressive difficulty in swallowing?
- Has there been progressive unintentional weight loss?
- Are there any other associated symptoms including nausea, bloating, feeling of fullness?

How Long has the Pain been Present and What are the Features of this Pain?

Much dyspepsia is recurrent. It is therefore important to confirm that the dyspepsia is a new episode. It is also important to exclude common causes of dyspepsia such as drug side-effects. Dyspepsia or pain in the epigastrium is common and usually has a benign cause.

Has there been any Bleeding?

Haematemesis requires emergency referral to hospital. Bleeding may also present in a well patient as melaena or blood in the stool. Cancer is a relatively uncommon cause of acute upper gastrointestinal haemorrhage, accounting for 2–5% of haematemeses. Malignant tumours of the stomach generally present with other upper gastrointestinal symptoms and with iron deficiency anaemia rather than acute bleeding. The presence of iron deficiency anaemia with dyspepsia warrants urgent referral for endoscopy. The most important benign tumour presenting with bleeding is a gastrointestinal stromal cell tumour.

Has there been Persistent Vomiting?

Vomiting is a common symptom and usually is self-limiting. The term 'persistent' is defined within the NICE guideline on *Dyspepsia: the management of dyspepsia in adults in primary care* as:

> the continuation of specified symptoms and/or signs beyond a period that would normally be associated with self-limiting problems. The precise period will vary depending on the severity of symptoms and associated features, as assessed by the healthcare professional. In many cases, the upper limit the professional will permit symptoms and/or signs to persist before initiating referral will be 4–6 weeks.

Has there been any Progressive Difficulty in Swallowing?

Dysphagia is the symptom of difficulty in swallowing, resulting in a delay in food reaching the stomach from the mouth. It can be separated into 'high' and 'low' dysphagia, which point to different causes. High dysphagia occurs predominantly in the pharynx or high oesophagus and is usually of neurological (e.g. stroke, Parkinson's disease) or anatomical (e.g. oropharyngeal malignancy, myasthenia gravis, cricopharyngeal spasm) origin. Low dysphagia may be caused by carcinoma of oesophagus or oesophageal junction, reflux disease or motility disorders (e.g. achalasia).

> **Box 11.4 Questions in a patient with dysphagia**
> - How long has it been present?
> - Where is the feeling of food sticking?
> - Has there been any unintended weight loss?
> - Is the dysphagia for fluids or solids?

How Long has it been Present?

This will give a clue as to how seriously important this symptom is. A short duration of symptoms (less than 4 months) is particularly worrying and needs urgent attention. A longer duration suggests achalasia.

Where is the Feeling of Food Sticking?

This may help identify 'high' from 'low' dysphagia as described above. However, not all patients can localise the site of dysphagia easily.

Is the Dysphagia for Fluids or Solids?

Cancers are more likely to present with a history of progressive dysphagia, first for solids and only later for liquids. These questions are only a guide and all patients with dysphagia require referral for further investigation.

Has there been Progressive Unintentional Weight Loss?

This is an important symptom, especially in the presence of other upper GI symptoms. Weight loss is discussed in detail in Chapter 4.

Are there any Other Associated Symptoms, Including Nausea, Bloating, Feeling of Fullness?

As noted above, these are other symptoms that may help to ascertain the seriousness of the dyspepsia, especially in the context of accompanying weight loss.

Examination in A Patient Complaining of Dyspepsia

The main reasons for conducting an examination of a patient complaining of dyspepsia are:

- to identify signs of anaemia
- to assess whether there is an epigastric mass
- to assess whether there is evidence of weight loss.

However, the absence of these signs should not preclude referral if worrisome symptoms are present.

Investigations in A Patient Complaining of Dyspepsia

The only valuable primary care-based investigation is a full blood count to identify iron deficiency anaemia. Many patients with dyspepsia are tested for *H. pylori* but its presence or absence should not delay referral for endoscopy if there are worrisome features.

Other Ways in which Patients may Present with Upper Gastrointestinal Cancers

Abdominal pain, as opposed to dyspepsia, is relatively rare in upper GI cancer. If the cause is a malignancy, then colorectal cancer is more likely (Chapter 6). Fatigue may complicate any cancer and is discussed in Chapter 4. Loss of appetite on its own is a difficult symptom but when it occurs in patients with gastric or oesophageal cancer, it is likely to be accompanied by weight loss and other gastrointestinal symptoms. It therefore often indicates widespread disease.

Delays in Diagnosing Upper Gastrointestinal Cancer in Primary Care

One of the aims of the GP in assessing patients with symptoms is to avoid delay in diagnosing cancer. A recent systematic review of delays in GI cancer identified the key issue of patient recognition of the seriousness of symptoms, with the overview summarised in Table 11.1.

The perception of symptom seriousness was often based on a personal or family history of similar symptoms and this could impact on delay. Fear of cancer can work in two different ways. The concern may lead to prompt attendance; alternatively, patients may be less likely to consult for fear of receiving bad news or having to undergo tests. Patients later diagnosed with stomach cancer delayed longer than those with oesophageal cancer.

When it is so complex for practitioners to differentiate between symptoms that are worrying and those that are not, it is easy to see how difficult it is for patients to recognise the seriousness of their symptoms. This does, however, present us with a challenge if we want to try to reduce the time

Table 11.1 Main delay factors by strength of evidence of dominant finding

	Overall assessment
Patient delay	
Non-recognition of symptom seriousness	Increases delay
Cancer site – stomach	Increases delay
Lower socio-economic status	Increases delay
Co-morbidity	Reduces delay
Presenting to hospital	Reduces delay
Male sex	No impact on delay
Fear	Inconclusive
Experiencing pain	Inconclusive
Older age	Inconclusive
Lower education	Inconclusive
Family history	Inconclusive
GP delay	
Initial misdiagnosis	Increases delay
Acid suppression treatment	Increases delay
Inappropriate/inaccurate tests	Increases delay
Previous negative test result	Increases delay
Cancer site – oesophagus	Increases delay
Female patient	Increases delay
Older patient age	Reduces delay
Lower patient socio-economic status	Reduces delay
Use of referral guidelines	Reduces delay
Co-morbidity	Inconclusive
Frequent patient attendance	Inconclusive
Use of rapid access endoscopy	Inconclusive

period of delay. It is easy to label GP delays as 'misdiagnosis' but it is fairer to say that there are considerable challenges for practitioners in assessing symptoms like dyspepsia, including evaluation of this symptom in the context of acid suppression therapy and previous negative test results. Such issues need to be clearly addressed within guidelines.

Investigations in Patients with Upper Gastrointestinal Symptoms

FBC, LFTs, ESR, CRP, *Helicobacter* serology

All these blood tests may be useful in patients complaining of the symptoms described in this chapter. However, negative results should not impact on the decision to refer for endoscopy, in the presence of other referral criteria. In particular, *H. pylori* status should not affect the decision to refer for suspected upper gastrointestinal cancer.

Barium Studies

Double-contrast barium studies were the investigation of choice until the 1980s when they were superseded by upper GI endoscopy, the latter being better particularly because of the ability to take biopsies. Barium studies are almost as sensitive as endoscopy for oesophageal cancer and advanced gastric cancer but are less sensitive in identifying early gastric cancer.

Endoscopy

Endoscopy allows the clinician to view the gastrointestinal tract and take biopsies and is now the gold standard investigation of the oesophagus and stomach. Most regions have direct primary care access to endoscopy services. Oesophageal cancer is diagnosed as a result of only 1% of total endoscopies carried out and gastric cancer as a result of 2%.

Pancreatic Cancer

Pancreatic cancer is relatively rare, with an incidence in Western Europe of 1 per 10,000 population per year. It is slightly more common in men and incidence rises with age. Risk factors include smoking, partial gastrectomy, dietary fat and a family history of pancreatic cancer.

The classic presentation is with painless progressive obstructive jaundice. This occurs particularly in carcinoma of the head of the pancreas. Cancers of the body or tail usually present with abdominal pain, anorexia and weight loss. Patients also frequently complain of epigastric or dull back pain. They may have the pale stools and dark urine of obstructive jaundice. Patients are usually jaundiced and may also look pale due to anaemia and show evidence of weight loss. Examination may reveal an epigastric mass.

In patients with obstructive jaundice, an urgent referral should be made, depending on the patient's clinical state. Alternatively, an urgent ultrasound investigation may be considered, if available. Other appropriate investigations include FBC, ESR and LFTs. Even in the absence of the classic features of obstructive jaundice, urgent referral would be recommended for patients who present with undiagnosed jaundice with weight loss and/or abdominal pain.

Hepatocellular Carcinoma

Hepatocellular carcinoma is relatively rare in developed countries but common worldwide. It accounts for 80–90% of all liver cancers. The disease is more common in parts of Africa and Asia than in North or South America and Europe.

Risk factors include being male, increasing age, cirrhosis, persistent hepatitis B or persistent hepatitis C infection. In the UK, over 90% of cases are associated with cirrhosis.

The symptoms are often non-specific and can include weight loss, pyrexia of unknown origin or feelings of fullness. Patients may have some right upper quadrant tenderness and an enlarged liver. Hepatocellular cancer should be considered in any patient with cirrhosis who is deteriorating clinically. Many of these patients will be under review at liver clinics and the cancer is more likely to be diagnosed there. Serum alpha fetoprotein may be elevated but it can be normal, so is of little value as a test in primary care. Definitive diagnosis is by liver biopsy.

Further Reading/Key References

Chen J, Rocken C, Malfertheiner P, Ebert M P 2004 Recent advances in molecular diagnosis and therapy of gastric cancer. Digestive Diseases 22:380–385

Delaney B C 1998 Why do dyspeptic patients over the age of 50 consult their general practitioner? A qualitative investigation of health beliefs relating to dyspepsia. British Journal of General Practice 48:1481–1485

Gullo L, Tomassetti P, Migliori M, Casadei R, Marrano M 2001 Do early symptoms of pancreatic cancer exist that can allow for an earlier diagnosis? Pancreas 22:210–213

Hohenberger P, Gretschel S 2003 Gastric cancer. Lancet 362:305–314

La Vecchia C, Tavani A 2002 A review of epidemiological studies on cancer in relation to the use of anti-ulcer drugs. European Journal of Cancer Prevention 11:117–123

Macdonald S, Macleod U, Campbell N C, Weller D, Mitchell E 2006 Systematic review of factors influencing patient and practitioner delay in diagnosis of upper gastrointestinal cancer. British Journal of Cancer 94:1272–1280

Mariscal M, Llorca J, Prietd D, Delgado-Rodriquez M 2001 Determinants of the interval between the onset of symptoms and diagnosis in patients with digestive tract cancers. Cancer Detection and Prevention 25:420–429

Tytgat G N J, Bartelink H, Bernards R et al 2004 Cancer of the esophagus and gastric cardia: recent advances. Diseases of the Esophagus 17:10–26

Chapter 12

Gynaecological Cancers

Clare Wilkinson and Roy Farquharson

Epidemiology

Cervical cancer

Cervical cancer is the second most common female cancer worldwide with a peak incidence at about age 50 years. In the UK, however, it is relatively rare, being the 10th most common female cancer. A GP will see a new case approximately every 10 years. In 2000, there were over 471,000 new cases diagnosed worldwide, with 288,000 deaths. Most cases (80%) occurred in the developing world, where women do not have access to screening programmes.

The incidence of abnormal cytology or histological evidence of cervical intraepithelial neoplasia (CIN) is substantially higher than that of invasive cervical cancer, as many of these precursor conditions spontaneously regress without treatment. Recent analyses and projection of UK trends suggest that 40% of untreated high-grade precursor lesions (CIN3) would progress to invasive cancer over the woman's lifetime. This equates to approximately 1% of women with CIN3 developing invasive cancer per year. A modelling exercise of this nature concluded that the cervical screening programme in the UK has prevented an epidemic of cervical cancer. Between 1988 and 1997, the incidence of cervical cancer fell by 42% in the UK. Incidence rates have also decreased steadily in the US over the past two decades. On the other hand, the cervical cancer incidence has not changed in developing countries unless they have 'progressed' to industrialisation and relative affluence. The WHO refers to the latter group as the 'middle-income' category. The highest incidences are found in some countries of Central and South America.

There is increasing evidence that high-risk types of the human papilloma virus (HPV 16, 18, 31, 33) cause invasive cervical cancer, with high-risk genotypes detected in virtually 100% of cancers.

Endometrial Cancer

Endometrial cancer is the most common malignancy of the female genital tract and the fifth most common female cancer behind breast, lung, bowel and ovarian cancer. A woman faces a lifetime risk of 1–2% of the disease and her GP will see a new uterine cancer around every 6–7 years. The average age at presentation is 60 years, since it occurs predominantly in postmenopausal women.

Oestrogen is a key factor in endometrial cancer, so any factor that leads to increased exposure to unopposed oestrogen also increases the risk of this cancer. There appear to be two types of cancer: an oestrogen-dependent type in younger peri- or postmenopausal women with a history of exposure to unopposed oestrogens and a non-oestrogen dependent (and more aggressive) type in older women.

Risk factors for endometrial cancer include nulliparity, late menopause, obesity, diabetes mellitus, unopposed oestrogen therapy and treatment with tamoxifen. Atypical endometrial hyperplasia is a precursor lesion, with the risk of it progressing to invasive carcinoma related to the severity of the cytological changes. For example, progression to cancer occurs in 1% of women with simple hyperplasia, 8% of women with atypical simple hyperplasia and 29% of women with atypical complex hyperplasia. Of those women who have atypical hyperplasia diagnosed from endometrial curettings, about one-quarter will have a well-differentiated endometrial carcinoma at hysterectomy.

Presenting Symptoms of Cervical and Endometrial Cancers

The most common presentations of invasive cervical cancer are with local symptoms such as irregular bleeding, especially postcoitally, and intermenstrual bleeding or foul-smelling discharge and back pain.

The most common presentations of endometrial cancer are with irregular bleeding during the perimenopause or postmenopausal bleeding or discharge. About 90% of women have bleeding or discharge as their only symptom. Women with more advanced-stage disease may have pelvic pressure or discomfort. However, although all women with postmenopausal bleeding need investigation, less than 10% will have endometrial cancer. Most of the rest will have a benign cause such as atrophy.

Clinical Examination

Cervical cancer

Bimanual vaginal examination of the pelvis and speculum inspection of the cervix are essential when a woman describes any of the symptoms listed above. Invasive cervical cancer may appear necrotic, ulcerated or as a protuberant 'cauliflower' lesion. It may be difficult to distinguish warty lesions from early malignancies of the cervix with the naked eye. If such a lesion is seen, there is no benefit in taking a cervical smear before referral. On pelvic examination, an invasive cancer is likely to have a discrete nature and often feels hard and craggy compared with the rest of the cervix.

Endometrial Cancer

Most women recognise the importance of postmenopausal bleeding and present to their GPs within 3 months. Although the symptom alone is enough to warrant urgent referral, bimanual vaginal examination and speculum examination in primary care is appropriate.

Investigation and Referral

The cervical and endometrial sections of the latest UK guidelines are summarised in Box 12.1. Symptoms such as alterations in the menstrual

---

Box 12.1   UK guidelines (2005) recommendations for urgent referral of possible cervical or uterine cancer

- Clinical features of cervical cancer on examination
- Postmenopausal bleeding in a woman NOT on hormone replacement therapy
- Postmenopausal bleeding in a woman taking tamoxifen
- Persistent intermenstrual bleeding even with a negative bimanual examination
- If an abdominal or pelvic mass is found which is not uterine fibroids, urological or of gastrointestinal origin, then urgent ultrasound and urgent referral should be considered (this recommendation also extends to ovarian cancer)

cycle, intermenstrual bleeding, postcoital bleeding, postmenopausal bleeding or discharge should prompt full pelvic examination and speculum examination of the cervix. Any unexplained abdominal symptoms should also prompt a full vaginal examination and abdominal palpation to exclude pelvic pathology. When a woman taking hormone replacement therapy has postmenopausal bleeding. it should be stopped for 6 weeks; continued bleeding after this should be urgently referred.

Staging, Treatment and Survival

Cervical cancer

If left untreated, invasive cervical cancer generally advances by extensive local invasion and spreads via the lymphatic system. The prognosis of treated invasive cancer depends on the stage at the time of diagnosis. The prognosis is excellent after treatment for early-stage disease. Microinvasive (<3 mm) stage IA cervical cancer can be treated conservatively with conisation in women wishing to preserve fertility; otherwise, the treatment is simple hysterectomy. Stages IB and IIA are treated with either radical hysterectomy or radiotherapy. Chemoirradiation is the current treatment for stages IIB, III and IVA. Some clinicians also use this in stage IB patients having radiotherapy as their primary treatment. Novel treatments may include tumour-specific gene therapy and vaccination against oncogenic HPV types.

Endometrial Cancer

Treatment for this cancer has changed over the past few decades, towards an individualised approach using hysterectomy as a primary therapy, with adjuvant treatment depending on staging and histology.

Adenocarcinomas account for about 80% of endometrial carcinomas. Less common histological types include mucinous, papillary serous carcinoma, clear cell carcinoma, squamous cell carcinoma, undifferentiated carcinoma and mixed carcinomas. Most patients should undergo surgical staging; in very unfit patients clinical staging is performed. This process identifies most patients with extrauterine spread and therefore strongly influences treatment decisions. Total abdominal hysterectomy and bilateral salpingo-oophorectomy are usual surgical treatments, with adjuvant radiotherapy, chemotherapy and progestins depending on factors related to staging and co-morbidity.

Minimising Diagnostic Delays

For both cervical and endometrial cancer, the key issue in primary care is to recognise the importance of clinical examination in the presence of high-risk symptoms amongst women in the appropriate age groups. The combination of symptoms and signs should lead to urgent referral. Difficulties remain in ensuring accurate primary care diagnosis due to the lack of evidence regarding the predictive value of these clusters of symptoms.

Screening and Risk Management Programmes

Cervical cancer

Theoretical aspects of screening are covered in Chapter 3. This section concentrates on the clinical aspects. The object of screening is to identify and treat the precancerous precursor lesion, cervical intraepithelial neoplasia (CIN) or squamous intraepithelial neoplasia. The precursor lesions are asymptomatic and can only be detected through screening. CIN is easily treated and prevents invasive cancer in most cases. Therefore, the sequelae are those arising from colposcopy, biopsy and local treatment; these processes have minimal physical and psychological sequelae. In terms of local treatment, only cold knife cone biopsy requires a general anaesthetic; other treatments are carried out during colposcopic examination.

The standard screening test for cancer of the cervix is the Pap smear or cervical smear test. This is performed by speculum examination, allowing direct visualisation of the cervix. The smear is taken from the transition zone or at the junction of the squamous and glandular epithelium. A wooden spatula is rotated 360° and the scraped cells spread onto a glass slide with fixative applied. Most cervical screening tests are carried out in primary care settings.

Liquid-based cytology (LBC) is currently being introduced as an alternative to conventional cervical cytology testing in a number of developed countries with full screening programmes. This method is designed to reduce the rate of inadequate tests and improve sensitivity. It involves using a brush-like device to obtain the sample, which is then suspended in buffer and processed so that a thin layer of cells is produced without contamination.

Women who are not infected with a high-risk HPV infection and have mild or borderline smear results are very unlikely to develop invasive cancer. Therefore, triage by HPV testing has been the subject of recent research but currently, HPV testing cannot be recommended for widespread use. Further information will become available from the UK-based TOMBOLA study during 2006 and the Dutch POBASCAM trial (Population Based Screening Study Amsterdam), which closes in 2007. These should provide evidence regarding whether cervical screening should be through a combination of HPV and cytology tests or be based on cytology alone.

Endometrial Cancer

There is no screening programme available for endometrial cancer since there is no test that can reliably identify precursor lesions.

Follow-up Practices

Follow-up after cytological abnormalities

The optimum management of mildly abnormal results is not clear and is the subject of a significant research programme in the UK, US and The Netherlands. Women who have borderline smears (also known as atypical or ASCUS) should be referred for colposcopy after three consecutive tests with this result. Women with one test reported as borderline changes in the endocervical cells should be referred for colposcopy. Ideally, one mildly dyskaryotic smear should generate a referral for colposcopy but it is an acceptable alternative simply to repeat the test. Although women should be referred and assessed, a 'see and treat' policy is often adopted in secondary care, to avoid overtreatment of CIN1. Patient choice over these management plans does not appear to have a marked impact on psychological outcome. Management of cytology suggestive of CIN2 or CIN3 or persistent milder abnormalities is by referral for colposcopy with histological sampling and treatment based on the histological finding. Women with invasive cells or cells indicating glandular neoplasia must be referred urgently for assessment.

Follow-up after Treatment for CIN

Commonly employed treatments for premalignant lesions include laser vaporisation or excision, cryosurgery, cold knife conisation, a loop electrosurgical excision procedure (LEEP) or simple hysterectomy. Some strategies such as LEEP combine diagnosis and treatment. All of these treatments are considered curative for CIN and are followed by a period of surveillance.

Further Reading/Key References

Comerci J, Goldberg G 2002 Current diagnosis and management of cervical cancer. Cancer Investigation 20: 524–530

Janicek M, Averette H 2001 Cervical cancer: prevention, diagnosis and therapeutics. Ca: a Cancer Journal for Clinicians 51: 92–114

Peto M, Gilham C, Fletcher O, Matthews F 2004 The cervical cancer epidemic that screening has prevented in the UK. Lancet 364: 249–256

Chapter 13

Brain Tumours

Kirsten Hopkins and David Kernick

Epidemiology

Primary brain tumours are rare, with around 4500 new cases each year. Brain metastases are more common than primary tumours, as they occur in 20–40% of patients with cancer. At the level of the individual GP, a new diagnosis of a primary brain tumour will occur among their patients approximately every 6–7 years. Malignant glioma is the most common primary brain tumour. It is progressively more common with increasing age. There is some geographical variation, although accurate interpretation is difficult; for instance, within England, the incidence is greater in the south than the north but this also correlates directly with the number of brain scanners. Gliomas are slightly more common in men than women.

Risk Factors

The aetiology of most primary brain tumours is unclear. A small percentage of patients will have a recognisable hereditary disposition, with gliomas occurring more frequently in individuals with neurofibromatosis and tuberose sclerosis. Rarely, two or more close relatives develop this uncommon malignancy, possibly representing inheritance of a yet unidentified gene.

Radiation can induce gliomas, with an increased incidence seen among children treated with radiotherapy for tinea capitis after the Second World War and after therapeutic pituitary radiation. Despite a furore of media attention and research, no association has been found with mobile telephone use. No aetiological factors are recognised in association with medulloblastoma or germ cell tumours.

Classification

Primary tumours

Gliomas arise from the glial supporting cells of the CNS. These are further divided as to their cell of origin, such as astrocytoma or oligodendroglioma. The overall 5-year survival for glioma is 18% but, in practice, clinicians divide primary brain tumours into two main groups.

First there are 'low-grade' tumours, comprising grades 1 and 2. Whilst this is a devastating diagnosis, many grade 1 tumours in children are completely cured. The median survival for patients with grade 2 tumours is approximately 5 years, with wide individual variation. Second, 'high-grade' tumours encompass Grades 3 and 4 tumours, also termed 'anaplastic astrocytoma/oligodendroglioma' and 'glioblastoma', respectively. High-grade tumours can develop either de novo or from transformation of a previously low-grade tumour. Grade 3 tumours will transform in time to grade 4 lesions, such that the prognosis is really a continuum, being an average of 2–3 years for patients with anaplastic astrocytoma and 10 months for individuals diagnosed with glioblastoma.

Meningiomas

Arising from the meninges, these tumours are usually benign and amenable to surgery. However, 5% are malignant. The overall 10-year survival for meningiomas is 80%.

Other Primary Tumours

Other primary tumours are rare in adults, occurring in fewer than 100 people in England and Wales each year. These include ependymomas, which arise from ependymal lining cells and may be low or high grade, medulloblastomas and other primitive tumours, germ cell tumours, malignant variants of meningeal tumours and other intracranial sarcomas. Patients generally present with similar symptoms to those with gliomas and successful treatment is hampered by the same challenges.

Primary Brain Tumours in Childhood

Brain tumours are the most common solid malignancy in childhood. The major differences in children are that tumours are most frequent in the posterior fossa and primitive tumours such as medulloblastoma and germ cell tumours are more common. High-grade gliomas, particularly in the brainstem, can occur and have a dismal prognosis.

Secondary Tumours

Secondary brain tumours are the most common cause of intracranial malignancy in adults. They may be the initial presentation of the patient's disease or there may be a prior history of malignancy. Cerebral metastases can occur with any systemic cancer but are more common with certain pathological types. Around half are metastases from lung cancer, small cell cancer having a particular predilection for cerebral spread. Approximately 20% follow breast cancer and a further 10% occur after a melanoma. Other primary sites with brain secondaries occurring fairly frequently are renal cell carcinoma, oesophageal or rectal cancers, whilst intracranial spread from ovarian or prostate carcinoma remains very rare.

Knowledge of the relative frequency of underlying primary sites helps in the choice of investigations when patients present with cerebral metastases. Clinicians often face dilemmas between, on the one hand, the expectations of the patient and their family (that comprehensive scans will be done to find and treat the primary cancer) and, on the other hand, the limited benefit that this may confer. In practice, clinical examination of the skin and breasts and a chest X-ray confirm the primary site in more than half the patients with little discomfort or resource implications.

Brain Tumour Diagnosis

Primary tumours of the CNS remain one of the hardest challenges for both primary care and oncologists. The diagnosis of these patients in primary care is hampered by several factors. Headaches are common yet primary brain tumours are rare. Indeed, GPs will see only a few of the latter in their entire career. Patients with secondary tumours may present to their oncology team rather than their GP, and have such a short survival that the GP is little involved. Symptoms of tumours may be diverse, depending upon their sites, and other much more common intracranial conditions such as cerebrovascular disease may confuse the picture.

Advances in neuroradiology have revolutionised the diagnosis of brain tumours. MRI is the investigation of choice as CT scanning at initial presentation misses around one tumour in 10. Access to brain scans is variable but often unsatisfactory and responsible doctors hesitate to overload systems when patients have uncertain symptoms. Radiological investigation is not without disadvantages. Apart from exposure to radiation with CT

> **Box 13.1   Summarised UK guidelines (2005 version) recommendations for urgent referral of possible brain and CNS cancer**
>
> - CNS symptoms, such as a progressive neurological deficit, new-onset seizures, headaches, mental changes, cranial nerve palsies or unilateral sensorineural deafness
> - Recent-onset headaches, with suspicion of raised intracranial pressure (the features that suggest raised intracranial pressure are vomiting, drowsiness, posture-related headache or tinnitus occurring in time with the pulse; blackouts or change in memory or personality are also possible)
> - A new, qualitatively different, unexplained headache that becomes progressively severe

scanning, studies in asymptomatic populations yield abnormalities ranging from 0.6% to 2.8%. These may cause considerable anxiety for the patient.

Symptoms

The UK guidelines, summarised in Box 13.1, suggest urgent brain scanning or specialist referral in several situations.

Presentation of Patients with Primary and Secondary Intracranial Tumours

Diagnosis begins with recognition of common symptom patterns. In general, the history triggers suspicion more frequently than examination findings. Clinical presentation can be a result of oedema around the tumour (particularly a feature of secondary tumours), direct mechanical pressure, obstruction of cerebrospinal fluid flow, or invasion or stretching of the meninges, leading to pain. Focal neurological symptoms more commonly occur in patients with primary tumours.

Headaches

The relationship between headache and tumour is always a concern for patient and doctor. This problem is magnified by the high frequency of headache as presented to primary care. Research on this topic has been limited by small sample sizes, a wide range of estimates, retrospective recall bias, specialist centre focus and conflation of acute and chronic presentations. This makes it very difficult to provide reliable figures for guidance.

In a 3-month period, 70% of the adult population will suffer from headache and 20% will have a significant problem. Up to 3% of GP consultations are for headache and 1 in 10 of these consultations will result in a referral to secondary care. Overall, around 30% of neurological referrals are for headache.

However, headache may be the initial symptom of a brain tumour. Around 70% of brain tumour patients describe a headache at some point during the course of their illness. At presentation, these figures are a little lower, being between a quarter and a half depending on the particular setting of the study. More importantly from a clinical perspective, the incidence of headache as a first and *isolated* presentation is much lower, at 2–16%. One prospective study suggested that isolated headache lasting over 10 weeks will only exceptionally be due to a tumour. One patient in 1500 of a primary care population presenting with isolated headache (and 1 in 150 of a secondary care population) will have significant pathology. Once primary headache (of which migraine is the most likely) is excluded then the risk becomes higher, at around 1 in 25, again for isolated headache. Severe headache with confusion occurring after an aeroplane flight can be a symptom of raised intracranial pressure.

Epilepsy

Seizure is the next most common presenting symptom of brain tumours, occurring in around 21% of patients, with 12% of first seizures being due to brain tumours. In a quarter of these patients the diagnosis of a tumour is delayed by 6 months or more, because of late presentation by patients or GPs not recognising the symptoms as epileptic. Furthermore, up to a quarter of patients with a seizure and a brain tumour have an initial negative CT scan. With tumours, seizures are generally recurrent, around 70% of patients having a subsequent seizure within the next 6 months.

Seizures arising from a brain tumour may be focal, partial complex, grand mal, temporal lobe attacks of altered taste or smell or 'déjà vu', or sensory epilepsy. Focal seizures are more common with primary tumours and generalised seizures with secondary ones but this is not a reliable rule. New-onset epilepsy in an adult is a prima facie indication for a brain scan, and major complaints have been upheld where this has not been done.

Confusion/Change in Cognitive Function

Patients with raised intracranial pressure may become obtunded, answering slowly, although in the early stages still correctly, to simple questions. It is obviously easier to identify this as pathological if the patient is well known to the doctor; if not, asking a relative if they have noticed a change in their personality is usually helpful. In more advanced stages, the patient may appear demented but usually an accompanying headache will alert the practitioner to the correct diagnosis.

Psychotic Behaviour/Change in Personality

These presentations are well recorded in the literature and do occur occasionally but are rare in comparison with the rather duller ones mentioned above. Anecdotes abound of the vicar's wife offering sexual favours to all parishioners and gentlemen with frontal lobe tumours blowing money in the belief that they are millionaires. Apathy is more common and the differential diagnosis includes depression. Once again, pre-existing knowledge of the patient is helpful and a history from relatives is mandatory.

Focal Symptoms

Focal neurological symptoms usually occur with solitary tumours and depend on the site of brain involved. The following are relatively common: hemiparesis; dysphasia and hemianopia.

Regarding hemiparesis, patients with disease at or adjacent to the motor cortex commonly present with unilateral weakness, with or without other symptoms such as sensory inattention and dysphasia. In primary care, such neurological loss is much more commonly from cerebrovascular disease than a brain tumour. It is rarely possible to distinguish whether an apparent stroke is due to a tumour at the first presentation. A history of progressive deficit over time, focal seizures, onset in younger patients without cardiovascular risk factors or a past history of malignancy should raise suspicion of a tumour. In any case, a suspected stroke requires immediate admission to hospital and the hospital team will perform a scan.

Dysphasia can occur alone or, more commonly, with a right hemiparesis. It almost inevitably signals disease in the motor speech area of the dominant hemisphere (usually left, even in left-handed individuals). Expressive dysphasia is immensely distressing for patients, and even more so when the underlying tumour means an early death is to be expected. Dysphasia is a particularly poor prognostic feature in patients with brain tumours, possibly because distress means that patients abandon treatment sooner.

Regarding hemianopia, patients with tumours in the posterior parietal region or occipital lobes commonly develop visual field defects. Recognition of these is relatively easy; there is usually a history of bumping into things and bruises or motor accidents to prove it. The classic problem is patients with a right hemianopia who drive out in front of traffic at roundabouts. Left hemianopia is safer: you merely destroy all the wing mirrors on parked cars on your nearside! Confirmation is straightforward with visual field testing.

Aspects of Presentation in Children

Brain tumours in childhood occur more usually in the posterior fossa, leading to hydrocephalus. This is associated with vomiting, increasingly severe headaches, ataxia and episodic loss of consciousness. This is a medical emergency but difficult, since the primary care differential diagnosis in sick young children is wide. Certain symptoms should give a clue, for example a history of the child holding their head awkwardly or with a torticollis. Headaches are not uncommon in children but a new headache, especially with any associated symptom, warrants investigation. Many children are referred late or even when moribund, a particular tragedy as many paediatric tumours are curable at an early stage, so it is difficult to reach any other conclusion than to recommend urgent referral of all children with worrisome symptoms.

Older children may present with brain tumours in the same ways as adults, reflecting increasing disease in the cerebral hemispheres but again, the low incidence of these tumours in adolescents sometimes delays recognition.

Further Reading/Key References

Grant R 2004 Overview: brain tumour diagnosis and management. Royal College of Physicians Guidelines. Journal of Neurology, Neurosurgery and Psychiatry 75: 18–23

King M, Newton M, Jackson G et al 1998 Epileptology of the first-seizure presentation: a clinical, electroencephalographic and magnetic resonance imaging study of 300 consecutive patients. Lancet 352:1007

Suwanwela N, Phanthumchinda K, Kaoropthum S 1994 Headache in brain tumour: a cross-sectional study. Headache 34:435–438

Vazquez-Barquero A, Ibanez F, Herrera S et al 1994 Isolated headache as the presenting clinical manifestation of intracranial tumours: a prospective study. Cephalalgia 14:257

Chapter 14

Childhood Cancer

Keith Sibson

Epidemiology

Cancer in childhood is very rare. Although there may have been a slight recent increase in incidence, in the UK only one child in 500 can be expected to develop a cancer before the age of 15 years: this equates to 1500 new cases per year in the whole country. Most GPs will encounter only a handful of cases in the whole of their career.

Risk Factors

In contrast to adults, the vast majority of cases of childhood cancer have no obvious cause. Large population studies have not identified any major contributory environmental factor, either before or after birth, although many theories exist. In addition, with a few notable exceptions such as retinoblastoma or Li Fraumeni syndrome, there is usually no family history of cancer. Siblings of children with cancer have roughly twice the chance of developing a malignancy in childhood themselves (i.e. 1 in 250), although for identical twins the risk is higher, rising to 1 in 4 for acute lymphoblastic leukaemia.

A number of genetic conditions carry an increased risk of developing a malignancy in childhood (Table 14.1). In the main, the families of such children will be only too aware of these associations and will usually present early. The degree of suspicion is so high in these children that any concern of the possibility of a new malignancy should prompt immediate referral to the paediatric service.

Table 14.1   Predisposing conditions for childhood cancer

Condition	Cancer type
Down's syndrome	ALL, AML
Neurofibromatosis	Fibrosarcomas, CNS tumours, phaeochromocytomas, juvenile myelomonocytic leukaemia
Tuberous sclerosis	CNS tumours, renal cell carcinomas
Fanconi's anaemia	Leukaemia, myelodysplastic syndrome, cancers of head/neck/oesophagus/liver/GU system
Wiskott–Aldrich syndrome	Leukaemia, lymphoma
Ataxia telangiectasia	Leukaemia, lymphoma, CNS tumours, thyroid carcinoma, gastric carcinoma
Xeroderma pigmentosum	Malignant melanoma, basal cell carcinoma, squamous cell carcinoma, fibrosarcoma
Dyskeratosis congenita	Hodgkin's disease, pancreatic carcinoma, squamous cell carcinoma
Bloom syndrome	Leukaemia, lymphoma, GI carcinoma
Beckwith–Wiedeman syndrome	Wilms' tumour, adrenal carcinoma
Von Hippel–Lindau syndrome	Haemangioblastoma, phaeochromocytoma

Presentation of Childhood Cancer

The presenting symptoms and signs of childhood cancer can be very similar to those seen in much more common childhood illnesses, most notably the ubiquitous viral infections, making it hard to pick out the few cases that require further investigation. A delay in diagnosis of several weeks to months (occasionally even years in the case of low-grade brain tumours) from the point of first contact is not uncommon.

Such a delay may have catastrophic medical consequences, for example in the case of a mediastinal mass being misdiagnosed as asthma. More commonly, a moderate delay does not impact adversely on the prognosis and long-term outcome of treatment. However, this can be difficult for parents to accept and may reduce trust in their GP. This is then compounded by the family building up a close relationship with the paediatric oncology team and shared care services. Even when the treatment is outpatient based, the child and their family still have frequent hospital visits, as well as open access to the local paediatric ward and specialist advice with the tertiary centre over the phone. As a consequence, the family may have no contact with their GP throughout the child's treatment.

For the child who later requires palliative care, this becomes particularly relevant, as most children dying of cancer these days are cared for at home, preferably with close involvement of their GP. After the child has died, the family quickly lose contact with the hospital and may require continuing long-term support closer to home. Even without this scenario, it is clearly not desirable for there to be a breakdown in relationship between a family and their GP.

How, then, does one swiftly make the diagnosis in the very few, without overinvestigating the very many?

Specific Cancers

Three groups of cancers make up the majority of childhood cancers: leukaemias/lymphomas, CNS tumours and bone/soft tissue tumours (Box 14.1). Two other clinical scenarios are relatively common: abdominal masses (rare, but cancer quite likely) and lymphadenopathy (common and cancer unlikely). These are described after the three main tumour groups. Lymphadenopathy in adults is covered in Chapter 4.

Leukaemia

Approximately one-third of paediatric malignancies are acute leukaemias, of which the most common form is acute lymphoblastic leukaemia (ALL)

Box 14.1 Relative proportions of different childhood malignancies			
Leukaemias	32%	**CNS tumours**	24%
ALL	26%	Astrocytoma	10%
AML	5%	Primitive neuroectodermal tumours	5%
Others	1%	Others	9%
Lymphomas	9%	**Soft tissue sarcomas**	7%
NHL	5%	Rhabdomyosarcoma	4%
Hodgkin's	4%	Others	3%
Neuroblastomas	7%	**Wilms' tumours**	6%
Bone tumours	4%	**Retinoblastomas**	3%
Germ cell tumours	3%	**Epithelial tumours**	3%
Hepatoblastomas	1%	**Others**	1%

with the remainder almost all being acute myeloid leukaemia (AML). The peak age for diagnosis of ALL is 2–3 years. The clinical features arise from a rapidly proliferating malignant clone (of an immature or mature haematopoietic cell) within the bone marrow. This process quickly 'takes over' the bone marrow, hence preventing normal haematopoiesis from taking place. This results in varying degrees of thrombocytopenia, anaemia and leucopenia, the effects of which are shown in Box 14.2.

As well as the above symptoms, bone pain (either localised to one point or widespread) is common and is due to expansion of the bone marrow cavity with leukaemic cells. These cells secrete cytokines which frequently cause intermittent fever. They also 'spill out' into the blood and tend to aggregate in lymph nodes, liver and spleen, causing lymphadenopathy and hepatosplenomegaly. If a child has any of the above features, a full blood count and blood film should be performed on the day they are seen (with a coagulation screen if there is bleeding or bruising). Leukaemia in the presence of a completely normal blood count (while reported) is incredibly rare and will reveal itself if repeat samples are taken.

The question of whether to seek for an underlying leukaemia in children with recurrent minor infections is tricky. Many children diagnosed with leukaemia have a history of recent recurrent infections, but this is probably coincidental rather than caused by the leukaemia. It is entirely reasonable not to take a full blood count in a child with a run of minor infections over the winter months or shortly after starting nursery. Equally, a normal result may provide reassurance to a particularly worried parent in such a situation. This is one of those times when there is no right answer. However, if the decision is made not to do a blood test, a thorough history

---

Box 14.2   Bone marrow failure

- *Thrombocytopenia* – easy bruising, spontaneous petechiae, recurrent epistaxis and gum bleeds
- *Anaemia* – tiredness/lethargy, pallor, tachycardia, cardiac failure if severe
- *Leucopenia* – severe/persistent infection

Box 14.3   Common presenting features of leukaemia

- Signs of bone marrow failure (see above)
- Unexplained fever
- Unexplained bone pain (irritability in young child)
- Widespread lymphadenopathy
- Hepatosplenomegaly

and examination need to be carried out, and recorded, to exclude any of the clinical features mentioned above.

More rarely, aggregations of leukaemia cells can occur at other sites in the body, in particular the central nervous system, chest, abdomen, testes and skin (where they are called chloromas). CNS leukaemia presents with symptoms and signs similar to those found in brain (or occasionally spinal) tumours and is discussed in more detail below.

Leukaemia Presenting as a Mediastinal Mass

T-cell leukaemia (or lymphoma) can cause an anterior mediastinal mass, as T-cells mature in the thymus. This is a medical emergency as these tumours are rapidly proliferating and can progress from being asymptomatic to life threatening within 48 hours. The cardinal signs are:

- dry cough
- wheeze and/or respiratory distress (particularly when lying down)
- superior vena cava obstruction (facial swelling and redness, distension of head and neck veins, headache, dizziness, reduced level of alertness).

This is an easy diagnosis to miss, as respiratory symptoms are so common with childhood infections. The superior vena cava obstruction may be very subtle. In addition, steroids are a very effective treatment for leukaemia or non-Hodgkin's lymphoma and if they have been used to treat presumed asthma, the signs may be masked for a while. It is therefore necessary to consider this diagnostic possibility; indeed, the paediatrician's mantra states that every patient presenting with their first episode of wheeze should have a chest X-ray before starting treatment.

Although T-cell leukaemia or non-Hodgkin's lymphoma causes the most dramatic presentation of a mediastinal mass, a range of other tumours can also present at this site, most notably Hodgkin's disease (where there may be the classic B symptoms of weight loss and night sweats present as well) and neuroblastoma (discussed in more detail below). Abdominal masses are more commonly mature B-cell leukaemias. They are particularly found in the region of the terminal ileum, where they can cause intussusception or mimic an inflamed appendix. Clearly, each of these conditions requires immediate referral to hospital.

CNS Tumours

As a group, brain tumours make up 25% of childhood malignancies. There are many different histological subgroups, the most common being

> **Box 14.4   Unusual presenting features of leukaemia**
>
> - *CNS* — cranial nerve palsies, seizures, raised intracranial pressure, headache, irritability, abnormal neurology
> - *Mediastinal mass* – respiratory distress, wheeze, cough, SVC obstruction
> - *Abdominal mass* – intussusception, 'appendicitis/appendix mass'
> - *Testes* – painless, hard, testicular enlargement
> - *Skin* – chloromas

astrocytomas and primitive neuroectodermal tumours (or medulloblastomas). The presenting features are dependent upon the site, the rate of tumour growth and the age of the child. For example, a teenager with a high-grade brainstem glioma may present early with rapidly evolving cranial nerve palsies. In contrast, low-grade tumours in the posterior fossa can grow to a remarkably large size before being detected in an infant whose sutures have yet to fuse.

The most common site is the posterior fossa, accounting for around half of all CNS tumours in childhood. Here they commonly cause cerebellar impairment and obstructive hydrocephalus. Supratentorial tumours may cause seizures or focal neurological impairment referable to their exact site. Brainstem tumours cause isolated or multiple cranial nerve palsies and damage to the long tracts. In each case, raised intracranial pressure can ensue and can even be the presenting feature. When this occurs, it constitutes a neurosurgical emergency requiring immediate referral for imaging and intervention. Similarly, although rare, if a child presents with loss of continence or weakness or impaired sensation in the lower limbs, an urgent MRI scan should be done to rule out a spinal cord tumour.

The precise symptoms and signs of brain tumours vary dramatically with age. Older children present in a very similar way to adults, but younger children find it difficult to describe abnormal sensations and signs may be more subtle. Infants with brain tumours frequently present in a very non-specific manner (e.g. vomiting, poor feeding, irritability) which can fool even the best GP. However, they also possess their own collection of signs which, if present, make the diagnosis a whole lot easier. Boxes 14.5–14.7 give age-appropriate symptoms and signs of brain tumours that should prompt an urgent referral for imaging and paediatric assessment.

Bone and Soft Tissue Tumours

Osteosarcomas and Ewing's sarcomas make up most of the bone tumours in childhood. Both cause either localised pain or a mass, or a combination

Box 14.5   Features of brain tumours in older children

- Headache worse on waking/lying down/straining
- Early morning vomiting
- New-onset seizures (particularly if focal)
- Change in behaviour or academic performance (not related to adolescence!)
- Cranial nerve palsies/visual disturbance
- Ataxia/nystagmus
- Focal weakness/change in sensation
- Unusual endocrine effects

Box 14.6   Features of brain tumours in younger children

- Any of the above
- Recurrent headaches of any description
- Recurrent vomiting if commoner causes excluded

Box 14.7   Features of brain tumours in infants

- Rapidly increasing head circumference (crossing two or more centile lines)
- Developmental regression (or delay following previously normal development)
- Squint, nystagmus or loss of red reflex
- Torticollis (tilted head position to overcome squint)
- Facial asymmetry (possible facial nerve palsy)
- Hand preference before first birthday (indicates hemiparesis)
- Loss of balance in sitting position (if previously stable)
- Persistent vomiting if commoner causes excluded/treated
- Persistent irritability/lethargy/poor feeding if commoner causes excluded

of the two. Osteosarcomas commonly present in adolescence and usually affect the femur, tibia or humerus. They metastasise to other bones and lung. Ewing's sarcomas tend to occur in the pelvis, femur, humerus and rib, with metastases involving lung, bone, pleura and bone marrow. Fever is an uncommon presenting symptom.

Rhabdomyosarcomas are the most common soft tissue sarcomas in childhood. They can arise at any site where primitive mesenchymal tissue has developed. The most common site is the head and neck, next the genito-urinary system and then the extremities. The superficial tumours present as a painless enlarging mass, but the deeper lesions can cause a variety of symptoms depending on their site, such as proptosis, nasopharyngeal blood-stained discharge and haematuria. Systemic signs are unusual, although again there may be bone marrow involvement.

In essence, the message is simple: any child with a new or enlarging bony or soft tissue mass requires referral for consideration of a diagnostic biopsy. In addition, any child with persistent bone pain (irrespective of whether a mass can be detected) deserves an X-ray, along with a full blood count and blood film to rule out leukaemia.

Abdominal Masses

Intra-abdominal masses can become huge before being detected. This is because:

- they are often painless
- they change the shape of the abdomen very gradually such that parents do not notice
- sometimes busy doctors do not examine the abdomen if the complaint is not directly referable to it – which is often the case.

Most such tumours occur in young children and in infants the only symptom may be irritability. Hence, if you have an irritable infant in your surgery without a firm diagnosis, it is worthwhile carefully examining the abdomen. The most common intra-abdominal masses are neuroblastomas, Wilms' tumours and B-cell non-Hodgkin's lymphomas.

Neuroblastomas

These occur at any site where sympathetic tissue is present and grow at a very variable rate from patient to patient. Almost all are diagnosed by the age of 2 but occasionally they can occur in older children, even young adults. Usually the primary tumour is a painless hard mass within the abdomen, arising from the adrenal gland. However, these tumours frequently also cause systemic effects (due to catecholamine release) such as fever, hypertension, irritability, weight loss, anaemia, and bone or joint pain. The latter can often be mistaken for an irritable hip before the primary tumour comes to light. Less commonly, respiratory symptoms due to a posterior mediastinal mass may occur and intraspinal disease can cause cord compression. Skin involvement sometimes can cause periorbital discolouration or the so-called 'blueberry muffin' effect in young infants. Finally, an autoimmune phenomenon may lead to cerebellar toxicity and is manifest as the 'dancing eye syndrome'. These names aptly describe the appearances and, when present, really cannot be missed.

Wilms' Tumour

These always arise from the kidneys and have far fewer systemic effects. They therefore usually present as an abdominal mass. In a minority, the first feature is painless haematuria. Irritability may again be a feature, due to hypertension or a low-grade intermittent fever. These tumours are associated with several conditions, such as Beckwith–Wiedeman syndrome, hemihypertrophy, aniridia and genitourinary anomalies. About 1 in 100 cases has a close family member with the same tumour. However, most children with Wilms' tumours have no significant past medical or family history and look strikingly well.

B-Cell Non-Hodgkin's Lymphoma

As with mature B-cell leukaemias, these tumours commonly present in the abdomen. In particular, they mimic appendicitis and can stimulate intussusception to occur. They are therefore often diagnosed by the paediatric surgeons at operation. Earlier clues to diagnosis might be signs of bone marrow failure, an abnormal blood film, generalised lymphadenopathy and hepatosplenomegaly.

Lymphadenopathy

Lymphadenopathy is a common presenting feature of lymphoma (and, less so, of leukaemia). It is also a very common finding in children with upper

Table 14.2   Lymphadenopathy in children: pointers to the diagnosis

Lymphomas	Reactive (infective)
Painless	Usually painful
Continue to grow	Rapidly grow and then gradually shrink
May be widespread	Usually localised
May be associated with: weight loss/night sweats/other masses	Associated with infection No night sweats/other masses

respiratory tract infections. The features that help to distinguish one from the other are listed in Table 14.2.

Summary

This chapter has highlighted the main presenting features of the commoner childhood malignancies. Some are obvious, but many are subtle and there is much overlap with minor conditions. In most cases where the symptoms are non-specific, a thorough examination and regular review will pick up the telltale signs. At times it is necessary to perform a blood test (when considering leukaemia), a urine dipstick (looking for haematuria) or an X-ray (in the child with isolated bone pain). However, all other investigations should be done within the context of an urgent referral to hospital. Paediatricians are happy to see children with features of a possible malignancy who prove to have something less significant. And, of course, parents will almost always desire a paediatric opinion if their child has unexplained symptoms. So, if in doubt, it is right to refer, and usually the sooner the better.

Further Reading/Key References

Greaves M 2002 Childhood leukaemia. British Medical Journal 324: 283–287
Pinkerton C R, Cushing P, Sepion B 1994 Childhood cancer management: a practical handbook. Chapman and Hall, London
Voute P A, Barrett A, Stevens M C G, Caron H N (eds) 2005 Cancer in children: clinical management. Oxford University Press, Oxford

Chapter 15

Haematological Malignancies

Jonathan Wallis and Pippa Harris

Epidemiology

Non-Hodgkin's lymphoma, leukaemia and myeloma are each in the 'top 20' most common malignancies. Taken together, they account for around 7% of new cancers. This percentage makes them the fifth most common malignancy overall. Thus, a full-time GP will encounter a new haematological malignancy approximately every 2 years. They may also encounter myelodysplasia, myeloproliferative disorders and other less aggressive diseases.

Terminology

Bone marrow stem cells may mature into lymphoid or myeloid cells.* Myeloid cells include neutrophil, basophil or eosinophil granulocytes, monocytes, erythrocytes and megakaryocytes. Clonal disorders are a proliferation of cells derived from a single aberrant cell, which has lost the normal controls of cell proliferation or programmed cell death. A simple classification of clonal diseases of haemopoetic cells is shown in Boxes 15.1 and 15.2.

Haematological Cancer Presentation

Patients with these diseases can present with:

- localised symptoms and signs such as enlarged nodes or spleen or bone pain

---

* We promise to use the expression 'bone marrow' as rarely as possible. Honest. The difference between GPs and haematologists is that bone marrow excites the latter and stupefies the former.

Box 15.1   Lymphoid proliferations

Acute lymphocytic leukaemia (ALL). A proliferation of immature lymphoid cells (lymphoblasts) mainly found in the blood and marrow. This is most common in pre-teenage children with a peak incidence of 8 per 100,000 per year at the age of 4 years. The incidence then falls to a low level (0.5 per 100,000 per year) in adult life.

High-grade non-Hodgkin's lymphoma (NHL). A proliferation of rapidly dividing immature lymphoid cells, as with ALL but mainly found in solid collections, usually in lymph nodes but sometimes extranodal, e.g. in testis or stomach.

Hodgkin's lymphoma. A proliferation of immature lymphoid cells with a large number of non-malignant inflammatory cells. It generally presents with localised nodal disease, most commonly above the diaphragm and is most common in young adults.

Low-grade non-Hodgkin's lymphoma. A proliferation of mature lymphoid cells chiefly present in enlarged nodes or spleen, often in the bone marrow and occasionally in the peripheral blood. It is generally found in the elderly.

Chronic lymphocytic leukaemia (CLL). A proliferation of mature lymphoid cells chiefly found in the blood and marrow, with enlarged nodes or spleen. This is also more common in the elderly.

Myeloma. A proliferation of mature antibody-producing B-lymphocytes in the bone marrow or, rarely, outside (extramedullary plasmacytoma) associated with production of a clonal immunoglobulin, detected as a paraprotein in the blood or urine.

Monoclonal gammopathy of uncertain significance (MGUS). This is a clonal proliferation of plasma cells producing a paraprotein where the infiltration of the marrow by plasma cells is at a very low or undetectable level.

A number of intermediate forms exist such as **lymphoplasmacytic lymphoma (or Waldenstrom's macroglobulinaemia),** which lies between CLL and myeloma, or **mantle cell lymphoma** or **hairy cell leukaemia,** 'half-way houses' between leukaemia and lymphoma.

- systemic and often non-specific symptoms such as weight loss and night sweats or skin problems
- symptoms of specific cytopenias such as fatigue or heart failure due to anaemia, bruising or purpura due to thrombocytopenia or infection secondary to leucopenia

---

Box 15.2 Myeloid proliferations

Myeloproliferative disorders. Excessive production of mature and functionally normal myeloid cells. These are more common with increasing age but may be diagnosed in young adults. Subtypes include: **polycythaemia rubra vera (PRV), essential thrombocythaemia (ET)** and **myelofibrosis (MF).**

Chronic myeloid leukaemia (CML) is now considered to be separate from the other myeloproliferative disorders because of its very distinct genotype (the Philadelphia chromosome). Those presenting with CML have increased numbers of mature and immature granulocytes in the blood, usually with a much enlarged spleen.

Chronic myelomonocytic leukaemia (CMML). Not to be confused with CML, this disorder is intermediate between myelodysplasia and myeloproliferative disorders. Monocytosis is invariable and the spleen may be enlarged.

Myelodysplasia. Production of functionally abnormal cells, which usually have poor survival. It typically presents with low blood counts of some or all of erythrocytes, granulocytes or platelets. It is very rare in young patients and the incidence increases with age.

Acute myeloid leukaemia (AML). Proliferation of immature myeloid cells or myeloblasts in blood and marrow. This may arise de novo or as a transformation of myeloproliferative or myelodysplastic disorders.

- an abnormal blood count performed as a routine screen or for some mild symptom or other disorder.

Lymphadenopathy

Lymphadenopathy may arise from a number of different cancers, so it is discussed in Chapter 4. Localised lymphadenopathy is found in HD and low- or high-grade NHL, while generalised lymphadenopathy is more common in low-grade NHL or CLL.

Splenomegaly (seen in NHL, ALL, CML, CLL and MPD) requires investigation and, unless there is evidence of liver disease or other clear cause, should be referred to a haematologist. If in doubt as to whether an abdominal swelling is a spleen, an ultrasound examination is simple and quick and also gives useful information about the liver and portal blood flow.

Bone Pain

Bone pain, typically back pain, may be due to myeloma. In a young child, persistent hip pain may be an early presenting feature of ALL with minimal changes in the blood but there are many alternative diagnoses, such as Perthes' disease. Bone or node pain after alcohol is a well-recognised but rare presenting symptom of Hodgkin's disease.

Does this Patient with Back Pain have Myeloma?

The ESR is typically raised in patients with myeloma producing a complete paraprotein. However, a low ESR does not exclude myeloma producing light chains only. These Bence-Jones myelomas (or the even rarer non-secretory form) often present at an advanced stage, with renal failure and/or hypercalcaemia (thirst, constipation and polyuria). Note that pure Bence-Jones proteinuria does not usually register on urine stick testing for protein.

If there is clinical reason to suspect myeloma, then request immunoglobulins and protein immunoelectrophoresis despite a normal ESR and request analysis of a spot urine for Bence-Jones protein.

Bone pain in myeloma is commonly due to vertebral collapse. This may be difficult to differentiate from osteoporotic collapse on plain X-ray.

Systemic Symptoms – Night Sweats

Clinically important night sweats are 'drenching'. The patient usually has to change their night clothes or the bed linen, or both. They are not associated with rigors but may be precipitated by a dose of paracetamol or an anti-inflammatory drug. Daytime sweats are less likely to be due to lymphoma. Night sweats may be seen with NHL, HD, CML and some more aggressive myeloproliferative disorders but are also seen with infections and other malignancies.

Skin Symptoms

Intractable itching may be the presenting feature of Hodgkin's disease. Itching is also an uncommon but well-recognised feature of myeloproliferative diseases when it is often worse after a hot bath. Painful red fingers (erythromelagia) or chilblain-like lesions on the feet may also be a presenting feature of essential thrombocythaemia. The pain responds rapidly to aspirin. Rarely, cold may induce purpura, or even skin ulcers, in patients who have a cryoglobulinaemia associated with NHL. Finally, infiltrating skin lesions can be seen in lymphomas (typically T-cell) and, rarely, AML or CML.

Cytopaenic Symptoms and the Full Blood Count

Almost every chapter in this book suggests a full blood count. Iron deficiency anaemia is described in Chapter 6, since colorectal cancer is the most common malignant cause. Normocytic or macrocytic anaemia is more common in haematological malignancies.

Thrombocytopenia

In thrombocytopenia, bleeding or bruising rarely occurs until the platelets are below $70 \times 10^9/l$ but a count of less than 150 is abnormal outside pregnancy. Isolated thrombocytopenia is more likely to be due to idiopathic thrombocytopenic purpura or drugs than to malignancy.

Neutropenia

Neutropenia is defined as below $1.7 \times 10^9/l$ neutrophils or below $1.3 \times 10^9/l$ in a patient of African origin. Recurrent infections usually only occur when the count is less than $1.0 \times 10^9/l$. Isolated neutropenia, as for platelets, is unlikely to be due to haematopoietic malignancy. Hypersplenism, immune neutropenia, drugs or viral infections are other possible causes.

Lymphopenia

Lymphopenia is common in many inflammatory states and may be persistent. It is seen in lymphomas but is not a very specific or useful pointer.

Miscellaneous Abnormalities on the Full Blood Count

Eosinophilia is sometimes seen in Hodgkin's disease, which can also cause a severe anaemia and a reactive thrombocytosis. Basophilia is marked in CML and may be seen in some other myeloproliferative cases but is rarely the main clue to the diagnosis. Monocytosis may suggest CMML or myelodysplasia but may also be seen in non-haematopoietic malignancy and chronic infective or inflammatory diseases, while absolute monocytopenia is an unvarying feature of the very rare hairy cell leukaemia.

Individual Disorders

Lymphomas

Non-Hodgkin's lymphoma accounts for 80% of cases, of which about half are high grade and half are low grade. Two-thirds of these present with nodal disease and one-third with extranodal disease. The incidence rises with age. Hodgkin's disease accounts for the remaining 20%, with a peak incidence in young adults.

High-grade Non-Hodgkin's Lymphoma

This can present almost anywhere in the body from bones to testis to stomach to brain. It is generally node based but about 30% are extranodal. The bone marrow may be involved although lymphoma cells are generally not seen in the blood. Systemic symptoms are common. The disease almost invariably progresses and the prognosis worsens with increasing bulk or spread of disease. Treatment, which should be started promptly, is nearly always by chemotherapy, often with radiotherapy to bulk or residual disease. Patients with localised disease have a good chance of a cure, perhaps 50–75%. Those with widespread and bulky disease have a 5-year survival of perhaps 25%. In addition to the degree of spread, the prognosis depends on the particular type of disease and, perhaps most importantly, the patient's age and co-morbidity. Palliative treatment with steroids alone or radiotherapy to bulk disease may be an option in the frail or elderly.

Hodgkin's lymphoma (HD)

This typically presents with neck lymph nodes, which may fluctuate in size, or with a mediastinal mass. The disease may be associated with marked systemic symptoms such as weight loss, sweats or itching. It may have a viral aetiology and Epstein–Barr virus can often be found in the Hodgkin cells in children and older patients but less often in young adults. Abnormal cells are not seen in the blood but reactive change, including anaemia, thrombocytosis, rouleaux and eosinophilia, is sometimes present. Treatment is usually with chemotherapy, though radiotherapy alone is still sometimes used in very early-stage disease. The prognosis is very good in young patients but less good in those over 50 years, for whom new regimes are being tried.

Low-Grade NHL

This comes in many forms but is usually widely spread in nodes and bone marrow at diagnosis. Survival at 10 years ranges from 50% for stage I to 25% for stage IV disease. If necessary, treatment is with fairly mild oral chemotherapy, or radiotherapy in the rare truly localised disease. However, observation alone may be appropriate if the disease appears stable and there are no symptoms related to bulk disease or from marrow suppression due to infiltration. Transformation to high-grade lymphoma can occur and may be difficult to treat. There is no evidence that early treatment improves the long-term outcome.

Chronic Lymphocytic Leukaemia (CLL)

This becomes much more common with increasing age. Many cases are diagnosed as a result of a chance blood count. Using lymphocyte markers on a peripheral blood sample, it is possible to show the presence of a clonal B-cell population even when the lymphocyte count is only slightly raised. Calling these cases CLL may be misleading and terms such as persistent lymphocytosis may be preferred.** In the absence of bulky nodes or evidence of marrow suppression (anaemia or thrombocytopenia), no treatment is needed and early treatment has not been shown to improve prognosis. Many cases are observed for years without change and die of other causes without ever needing treatment for the 'CLL'. Newer prognostic markers are being evaluated for their ability to identify those who will progress and might benefit from early treatment.

Other patients present with enlarged nodes and spleen or a very high lymphocyte count with marrow suppression. Treatment is usually recommended for these patients but it is not curative and the period of control is variable. An alkylating agent such as chlorambucil is traditional but newer and more powerful agents such as fludarabine, alone or in combination with other drugs, are being used more widely. CLL may be associated with reduced immunoglobulins and recurrent infections, particularly pneumonia and bronchitis. Treatment with long-term penicillin or regular immunoglobulin infusions may help.

Myeloma

Myeloma, like CLL, increases in incidence with age. Patients present with bone pain due to fractures, usually in the back, hypercalcaemia, renal failure, infections (typically pneumonia) or anaemia. Like CLL and low-grade NHL, there is no evidence that early treatment of disease is beneficial in the long term. Indications for treatment are damage to the bones or

---

** We are not advocating lying to one's patients. Clearly, one has to be as informative as possible. A good parallel is with basal cell cancer of the skin — isn't rodent ulcer a better expression?

suppression of the normal marrow, or damage to other organs from the paraprotein. Treatment controls the disease for a variable period but cure is very rare. Melphelan has been used for nearly 40 years. It is still a simple and effective treatment but in fitter patients use of alternative regimes followed by high-dose melphelan with autologous stem cell rescue has been shown to produce longer and better remissions. Mean survival after diagnosis for all patients has increased from around 24 months to 36 months. In those achieving remission, this may last over 5 years. Control of bony disease with oral or intravenous bisphosphonates has been a major advance in treatment.

MGUS and Indolent Myeloma

Low-level paraproteins are found with increasing frequency as age advances and with more sensitive laboratory equipment. They may be present in as many as 5% of those aged over 70 years and 10% of those over 80. The decision to investigate further depends on the patient's age and the level and type of paraprotein. As a general rule, if it is a chance finding without other evidence of plasma cell disease, an IgG paraprotein of less than 5 g/l does not need further investigation. In those under 65 years it is worth checking again after 6 months. With an IgG paraprotein level between 5 and 10 g/l, most haematologists would recommend observation without a bone marrow or other invasive testing. Full blood count, calcium and renal function should be checked and the paraprotein level repeated at 6–12 month intervals. Patients with over 10 g/l of IgG paraprotein should generally be investigated with a bone marrow and skeletal survey. Those with significant plasma cell infiltration of the marrow can be regarded as indolent or asymptomatic myeloma and should be followed carefully. IgA paraproteins may be important at a lower level; as a rule of thumb, multiply the result by two and then treat as for IgG paraproteins.

Levels of less than 5 g/l of IgM paraprotein are rarely of clinical significance but it is wise to check for anaemia, splenomegaly and lymph nodes, referring if they are present or if the paraprotein level is rising. Levels over 5 g/l may warrant further investigations. Very high levels may be associated with hyperviscosity syndromes (headache, confusion, bleeding problems) and it may even be difficult to take the blood. A few patients produce a cryoglobulin and may have cold-induced purpura or vasculitis.

About a quarter of patients with MGUS develop into myeloma if they live long enough (20 or more years). The chance of this is related to the original level of paraprotein. Transformation tends to occur suddenly, so regular follow-up of minor paraproteins is of little use.

Myeloproliferative Disease

Primary polycythaemia (PRV)

A raised haemoglobin may be due to primary polycythaemia or be secondary to lung or cyanotic heart disease, or to erythropoietin-producing renal tumours. A raised or high normal erythropoietin level is a good indicator that the polycythaemia is likely to be secondary rather than primary. Sometimes the total red cell mass is normal with a reduced plasma volume, so-called 'stress' polycythaemia, though stress itself has little to do with it (excess alcohol, coffee or diuretics may be involved).

Untreated, many patients with symptomatic primary polycythaemia die within a few years, mostly from thrombosis. This is probably due both to the increased haematocrit and to the abnormal platelets. Venesection is a practical and effective way of reducing the haematocrit to <45%. Most patients should also be on aspirin. Some may benefit from cytoreductive treatment with hydroxycarbamide (formerly known as hydroxyurea) but lingering concern remains that this may increase the long-term risk of leukaemic transformation. Overall, the prognosis of the disease is very good if treated.

Essential Thrombocythaemia (ET)

Patients may present with thrombosis, often stroke or, less commonly, with bleeding. Aspirin alone may be sufficient treatment in younger patients. In patients with a platelet count over $1000 \times 10^9/l$ or other risk factors for thrombosis (such as age over 60, smoking and diabetes), it is current practice to reduce platelet counts to normal or near normal with hydroxy-carbamide (hydroxyurea). The prognosis is also very good if treated.

Myelofibrosis

This is the least common of the myeloproliferative disorders, often present-ing with a large spleen, sometimes with high and sometimes low blood counts. Splenic infarcts may mimic pleuritic pain. The prognosis is mixed, with some patients being stable for many years while others progress more rapidly to a leukaemic state.

Chronic Myeloid Leukaemia (CML)

This is a genetically distinct disease that may present with fatigue, splenomegaly, sweats or even gout. The incidence increases linearly with age. Treatment has been revolutionised by the introduction of the oral agent imatinib, which specifically blocks the aberrant protein produced by the genetic mutation. Before imatinib, the mean prognosis was 3.5 years from diagnosis to death, with very few survivors beyond 8 years without marrow transplantation. Since the introduction of imatinib, average survival is over 5 years but may be much more.

Acute Myeloid Leukaemia (AML)

The incidence of AML increases exponentially with age. Presentation is normally with symptoms of anaemia or thrombocytopenia. The prognosis worsens with age. Under the age of 30 years, about 25% achieve a long-term remission or cure. Few patients over 60 survive more than 3 years and 90% of over-70s are dead within 12 months. The disease may be biologically different in the elderly, often developing from myelodysplasia (see below). Furthermore, elderly patients may not be fit for all or any of the treatment options. Acute promyelocytic leukaemia is a subtype of AML relatively more common in young patients that presents with troublesome, sometimes fatal, bleeding. This is a haematological emergency. If patients survive the initial phase then prognosis is quite good.

Myelodysplasia

Myelodysplasia is becoming increasingly common as the population ages. It may arise de novo or after chemotherapy for haematological and non-haematological disease. The bone marrow is taken over by a single clone of abnormal cells that produce low numbers of functionally defective cells. This results in peripheral cytopenias. The cells can undergo further mutations, leading to an overt leukaemic state. The subclassification breaks myelodysplasia down into milder forms, refractory anaemia and refractory anaemia with ring sideroblasts (acquired sideroblastic anaemia) and a more severe form, refractory anaemia with excess blasts, which merges with frank AML.

Acknowledgements

Our thanks to Professor S. Proctor and Dr P. Taylor for regional epidemiological information and to Dr G. Jackson and Dr M. Reid for helpful comments.

Further Reading/Key References

Cartwright R A, Gurney K A, Moorman A V 2002 Sex ratios and the risks of haematological malignancies. British Journal of Haematology 118:1071–1077

Chapter 16

Testicular Cancer
Richard D. Neal

Epidemiology

Although testicular cancer is the most common cancer in younger (18–35 year old) men, it is still a rare disease. It is rare in those aged less than 20 and increasingly uncommon above the age of 40–45 years (Fig. 16.1). There are about 2000 new cases per year in the UK and about 100–150 deaths. This equates to about one new case every 15 years for each full-time GP in the UK.

The incidence is slowly increasing (Fig. 16.2). About 40% of testicular cancers are seminomas and about 60% teratomas, although many of these are mixed tumour types. Less than 5% are lymphomas and these generally occur in older men.

Risk Factors

Many factors are thought to affect an individual's risk of developing testicular cancer; however, it is likely that the individual risks associated with many of these factors are small. These risk factors include developmental abnormalities, such as testicular maldescent and cryptorchidism. This risk applies for disorders of the other testis too. Inguinal and testicular problems in childhood also increase an individual's risk of cancer. These include mumps, orchitis, inguinal hernia, torsion and hydrocoele. Genetic conditions including true hermaphroditism, testicular feminisation, Mullerian syndrome and Klinefelter's syndrome also increase the risk. Individuals with previous cancer in the contralateral testis and with HIV/AIDS are also at increased risk. Even so, this increased risk is very small. A family history of testicular cancer may be relevant. Having a first-degree relative with the disease increases the risk an estimated sixfold. Inherited genetic factors may play a role in up to 1 in 5 cancers.

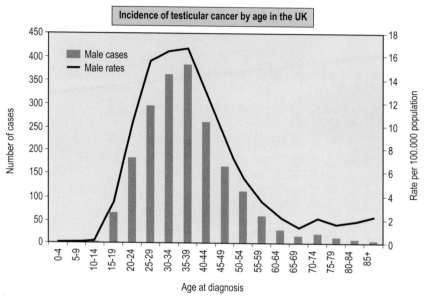

Figure 16.1   Incidence of testicular cancer by age in the UK (reproduced with permission from Cancer Research UK, Jan 2006. http://info.cancerresearchuk.org/cancerstats/types/testis/incidence/).

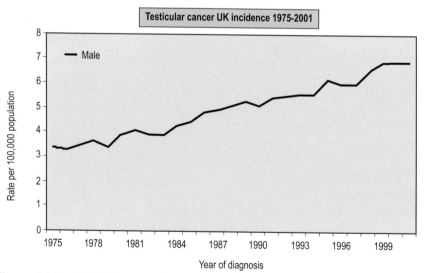

Figure 16.2   Testicular cancer UK incidence 1975–2001 (reproduced with permission from Cancer Research UK, Jan 2006. http://info.cancerresearchuk.org/cancerstats/types/testis/incidence/).

Presenting Symptoms

The most common presenting symptom of testicular cancer is a painless lump or swelling (>85%). The next most common presentation is an acute painful testis; this may represent torsion, bleeding or infarction as a result of the tumour. At presentation, 20–30% of patients experience a heavy dragging feeling or general ache. Cancer may occasionally present with symptoms that have previously been 'diagnosed' as recurrent epididymitis. A small number present with a hydrocoele. In a few the initial presentation is with symptoms of metastatic disease, including breathlessness, cough and haemopytsis; abdominal pain, lower back pain (if there is retroperitoneal spread affecting the psoas muscle or nerve roots); and infertility. Gynaecomastia may be present if the beta-human chorionic gonadotrophin is raised.

Patients may present with either a new discovery of a testicular lump or a lump that has increased in size relatively quickly. As a general rule, teratomas grow quickly and seminomas more slowly. Symptoms may also be presented as trivial secondary problems whilst consulting for a different primary reason. The man may simply be too embarrassed to voice his fears about his testicular symptoms.

Clinical Examination

Despite often high levels of embarrassment, and often an unfamiliarity with consulting, a thorough clinical examination is needed when a man reports a testicular symptom, however trivial. It is good practice to offer a chaperone, although this may often be declined.

A true testicular swelling is one that an examiner can get above when palpating (Fig. 16.3). It may be cystic or solid, and may be tender. The other testis must also be examined for comparison and to check for bilateral disease. If the patient has a hydrocoele (which transilluminates) or a haematocoele (which does not transilluminate), then the testis is within the swelling and a tumour cannot be excluded. Other causes of solid primary testicular masses include torsion, orchitis, testicular gumma and tuberculosis. Causes of masses that can be felt separate from the testis (but which may present as a 'lump') include epididymal cysts, acute and chronic epididymitis, torsion of hydatid of Morgagni and spermatocoeles. Important issues for the GP are to distinguish whether the 'lump' is a testicular lump or one arising from other scrotal tissues and to distinguish differences between one side and the other. Solid swellings affecting the body of the testis have a high probability (>50%) of being due to cancer.

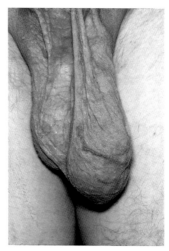

Figure 16.3   Testicular swelling (photo courtesy of Ian Daniels).

Box 16.1   Summarised UK guidelines (2005 version) recommendations for urgent referral of possible testicular cancer

- Any swelling or mass in the body of the testis
- In men with a scrotal mass that does not transilluminate, or if the body of the testis cannot be distinguished, an urgent ultrasound should be considered

---

In the presence of a testicular lump, examination of the chest (for chest signs and gynaecomastia), abdomen (organomegaly and for evidence of bulky nodal disease), and back and neck (supraclavicular lymphadenopathy) must be conducted for evidence of metastatic spread.

Investigation and Referral

The UK referral guidance is summarised in Box 16.1. It is very simple to follow.

Non-Urgent Referral

There is no need to urgently refer swellings outside the body of the testis. These can sometimes be managed by clinical diagnosis and empirical treatment or by non-urgent ultrasound and referral if needed. However, for many patients diagnosis and management can take place entirely within primary care.

Ultrasound

If local arrangements for urgent ultrasound examination permit, then this can be requested in parallel with an urgent suspected cancer referral. Swellings in men over 55 years, especially indeterminate ones, should be considered for ultrasound before urological referral, since the likelihood of malignancy is much lower.

Other Imaging

Further imaging is only probably indicated when more extensive disease is suspected and is therefore primarily a secondary care issue. A chest X-ray is needed if lung pathology is suspected and CT remains the treatment of choice for both disease staging and for assessment of response to treatment and ongoing surveillance.

Blood Tests

Non-seminomas have high levels of beta-human chorionic gonadotrophin, alphafetoprotein and lactate dehydrogenase and these are routinely checked in urology departments. They have little use in primary care diagnosis since all patients with swellings of the body of the testis should be referred urgently.

Staging, Treatment and Survival

For patients with a clinical diagnosis of testicular cancer on ultrasound, CT staging is usually undertaken prior to orchidectomy, after which a 'tissue diagnosis' can be made. Treatment options then depend upon the histology and spread of disease. Seminomas are especially radiosensitive tumours and teratomas are sensitive to chemotherapy. Courses of adjuvant chemo- or radiotherapy are sometimes also advised. Unlike many cancers, survival rates are good, generally in excess of 90%; this has increased significantly in the past three decades with improved treatments. Compared with most other cancers, patients with advanced disease still have a high rate of survival, albeit lower than patients with early localised disease. Overall survival worsens with age at diagnosis. So-called 'salvage chemotherapy' can be used to treat metastatic relapse and can be curative. Where treatments cause infertility, sperm may be banked, retaining the potential for biological fatherhood. Prosthetic testes are available and provide a good cosmetic result.

Minimising Diagnostic Delays

There is some evidence associating longer diagnostic delays with poorer outcomes. However, this body of evidence is relatively weak, given the excellent prognosis for even advanced disease. The only actions that clinicians can take to minimise delays are to be vigilant for testicular symptoms and refer for an urgent opinion or for an urgent ultrasound appropriately.

Testicular Self-Examination

Regular testicular self-examination has been advocated as a measure to facilitate earlier diagnosis of testicular cancer. Whilst there is no good evidence that this reduces mortality, regular testicular self-examination may lead to cancers being diagnosed at an earlier stage, with reduced morbidity and less invasive treatments. However, it may also cause anxiety and may lead to iatrogenesis as a result of 'lumps' being incorrectly found on routine self-examination.

Public understanding of testicular cancer, such as the age groups most at risk and the fact that treatment is invariably curative, is poor. The proportion of men who report regularly conducting testicular self-examination according to guidelines is small (about 20%). Health professionals should therefore consider promoting testicular self-examination, with some caution, for men aged 15 and above (Box 16.2).

Further Reading/Key References

Chapple A, Ziebland S, McPherson A 2004 Qualitative study of men's perceptions of why treatment delays occur in the UK for those with testicular cancer. British Journal of General Practice 54:25–32

Neal R, Stuart N, Wilkinson C 2005 Testicular cancer: seminoma. In: Clinical evidence. BMJ Books, London

DIPEx database of patient experience: www.dipex.org.uk

Box 16.2   Testicular self-examination instructions

- The best way to check for testicular cancer is to examine yourself once a month. A good time to do this is after a warm bath or a shower, when the scrotal skin is relaxed.
- Hold the scrotum in the palms of your hands, so that you can use the fingers and thumb on both hands to examine your testicles.
- Note the size and weight of the testicles. It is common to have one testicle slightly larger or which hangs lower than the other but any noticeable increase in size or weight may mean something is wrong.
- Gently feel each testicle individually. You should feel a soft tube at the top and back of the testicle. This is the epididymis which carries and stores sperm. It may feel slightly tender. Don't confuse this with an abnormal lump.
- You should be able to feel the firm smooth tube of the spermatic cord that runs up from the epididymis.
- Feel the testicle itself. It should be smooth with no lumps or swellings. It is unusual to develop cancer in both testicles at the same time, so if you are wondering whether a testicle is feeling normal or not, you can compare it with the other.
- Remember, if you do find a swelling in your testicle, make an appointment and have it checked by your doctor as soon as possible.

Source: www.cancerhelp.org.uk

Chapter 17

Head, Neck and Thyroid Cancers

William Hamilton

Epidemiology

Although these cancer sites are anatomically close to each other, they are very different in their risk factors and presentation.

Oral Cancer

Oral cancer is slowly increasing in incidence in the UK, accounting for around 1% of new cancers, with almost 3000 new diagnoses each year. It is almost twice as common in men as in women, reflecting the risk factors of smoking and alcohol. A full-time GP will only have a patient newly diagnosed approximately every 10 years or so. Furthermore, many patients are identified by dental services, with the GP having little input.

Risk Factors

Three main predisposing factors have been identified. Cigarettes and alcohol are both independent risk factors. The third factor is the use of pan-tobacco, a combination of betel leaf and other vegetable products. Pan-tobacco chewing is popular in people of South Asian extraction.

There is a recognisable premalignant phase in oral cancer, with the normal epithelium changing over a period of years. Three precancerous lesions are described: leukoplakia, erythroplakia and erythroleukoplakia (Fig. 17.1). Of these, erythroleukoplakia has the greatest potential for malignant transformation but is the rarest. The 2005 version of the referral guidelines for suspected cancer recommend urgent referral of unexplained

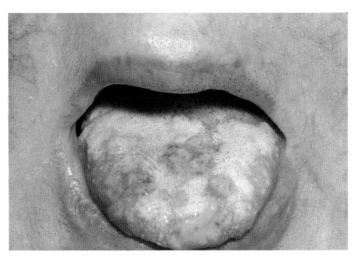

Figure 17.1   Erythroleukoplakia (photo courtesy of Ian Daniels).

red and white patches (more strictly, red *or* white) on the oral mucosa that are painful or swollen or bleeding.

Screening for oral cancer is not offered in the UK, though trials of screening in high-prevalence areas have yielded favourable results.

Oral Cancer Presentation

The cancer usually appears as an unhealing ulcer on the tongue, buccal mucosa or lip. It often has a deep, punched-out appearance, especially on the tongue. The ulcer is generally shallow when it is on the lip. Most of these presentations are obviously abnormal and are relatively easy for a GP to identify (even if they cannot be completely confident of the diagnosis). The referral guidelines recommend urgent referral for an unexplained ulcer or mass that has been present for 3 weeks or more. Cancers that are more difficult to diagnose are those that present as a lump or as a red raised patch on the buccal mucosa. Given that most patients with this type of abnormality have had their symptoms for months rather than weeks, it is usually easy for the GP to justify a referral to the 2-week clinic for investigation of suspected cancer. Some patients present with enlarged cervical lymph nodes and this topic is covered in Chapter 4.

Diagnosis at an advanced stage is depressingly common with oral cancer. The median delay from the first symptom until diagnosis is 3 months (with most of the delay being attributable to the patient). This figure has not improved over the last 40 years and nor has the proportion of patients presenting with advanced disease at diagnosis.

> **Box 17.1   UK guidelines (2005 version) recommendations for urgent referral of possible laryngeal cancer**
>
> - An unexplained persistent sore or painful throat
> - An unexplained lump in the neck (see Chapter 4)
> - Hoarseness persisting for more than 3 weeks – for urgent chest X-ray and ENT referral if X-ray is negative

Laryngeal Cancer

Laryngeal cancer is almost as common as oral cancer, with just under 2500 new diagnoses in the UK in 2000. The full-time GP will encounter a new diagnosis of laryngeal cancer less frequently than once in 10 years. It is even more a disease of males than oral cancer, with a sex ratio of over 4:1. Like oral cancer, laryngeal cancer is much more common in those who smoke.

Laryngeal Cancer Presentation

The most common symptoms are: a change in the voice, principally to hoarseness; local pain; neck swelling; and dysphagia. Stridor may be a late symptom. This is reflected in the recommendations encapsulated in the referral guidelines presented in Box 17.1.

Sore Throat

Sore throats are extremely common in primary care and many are persistent. No studies from primary care allow the calculation of a PPV of a persistent sore throat for laryngeal cancer but it must be considerably below 1%. A large American survey of 492 head and neck cancer patients concluded that no symptom other than hoarseness was helpful in the early identification of these cancers.

Hoarseness

This is also a relatively common symptom in primary care, although most consultations for hoarseness are in younger age groups. Infection is the usual cause. Almost all laryngeal cancer patients have some hoarseness, even those whose tumour is above the vocal chords.

A full-time GP will see approximately one patient over the age of 40 years with hoarseness each month. Given that this GP will see one laryngeal cancer each decade (at most), the PPV of hoarseness must be under 1%. The median duration of hoarseness by the time laryngeal cancer is diagnosed is over 3 months. Like oral cancer, most of this 'delay' can be attributed to the patient, as the median duration before it is reported to the GP is 2 months. Therefore, most of those patients whose hoarseness is due to cancer will already have had their symptom long enough by the first presentation to the GP to warrant urgent referral for investigation.

Of the malignant causes of persistent hoarseness, lung cancer is much more common than laryngeal cancer. That is why a chest X-ray is deemed the appropriate first investigation. It is, however, rare for lung cancer to present as isolated hoarseness.

Thyroid Cancer

This is even more uncommon, occurring only once (if at all) in a GP's clinical lifetime. It occurs in younger patients than most cancers, with a median age at diagnosis of 45 years. It is twice as common in women as in men. Occasionally, it may be part of an inherited syndrome, such as familial adenomatous polyposis or Gardner's syndrome. Medullary carcinoma of the thyroid is one of the tumours that make up multiple endocrine neoplasia, although only 20% of such tumours are part of such a syndrome, the remainder being sporadic. An abnormal gene for multiple endocrine neoplasia has been identified and reliable testing is available for family members. Prophylactic thyroidectomy is carried out in those found to carry the abnormal gene and this is usually performed in childhood.

The risk of thyroid cancer is greatly increased by external radiation, especially during childhood. This was one late effect of the Chernobyl nuclear incident, with an increase of up to 75 times the expected rate of thyroid cancer in regions affected by radio-active fallout.

Thyroid Cancer Presentation

Almost all thyroid cancers present with a nodule, usually painless. All such nodules warrant referral for fine needle aspiration. The only exception is anaplastic carcinoma (which makes up about 1% of all thyroid cancers), shown in Figure 17.2. It generally produces a larger mass – and the referral decision should be easy.

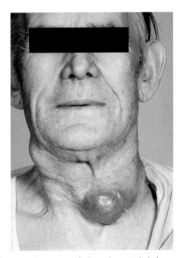

Figure 17.2   Anaplastic carcinoma of the thyroid (photo courtesy of Ian Daniels).

Further Reading/Key References

Epstein J, Zhang L, Rosin M 2002 Advances in the diagnosis of oral premalignant and malignant lesions. Journal of the Canadian Dental Association 68:617–621

Raitiola H, Pukander J 2000 Symptoms of laryngeal carcinoma and their prognostic significance. Acta Oncologica 39:213–216

Sherma S I 2003 Thyroid carcinoma. Lancet 361:501–511

Thomas G, Hashibe M, Jacob B et al 2003 Risk factors for multiple oral premalignant lesions. International Journal of Cancer 107:285–291

Van der Goten A 2004 Evaluation of the patient with hoarseness. European Radiology 14:1406–1415

Chapter 18

Case Histories

William Hamilton

These cases are relatively straightforward and are designed to be used in two different ways. Experienced practitioners may simply want to use them as debating points, whereas inexperienced GPs may want to be more formal in actually writing down an answer. They are based around a fictitious practice of 9000 patients and five doctors. Over a year, around 50 new cancers will be diagnosed in the practice but many more will have symptoms that may represent a cancer. The 50 cancers will be mostly lung, breast, colon, prostate and skin. However, I have included some cases from the rarer cancers, meaning there is a disproportion of atypical cancers. This is unavoidable.*

Several of the cases are based on real stories. In this respect, the Medical Protection Society were extremely helpful in allowing me access to their reports of cancer cases. I wish to thank them and the clinicians involved for allowing re-publication in an altered form. All names and identifying details have been changed twice, so any similarity to a real person is unintentional.

---

* As it happens, the practice is centred on an industrial estate with a (leaky) nuclear power plant, a dye factory and an asbestos works. The population largely ignore medical advice, are overweight and have diets consisting of heroic amounts of tobacco and alcohol.

Case history 1
Simon

The first week of January in general practice is always dreadful. The problem is New Year's resolutions – which are rarely to cease smoking. The surgery fills with people wanting their blood pressure and/or cholesterol checked. Simon, a 29-year-old postman and father of two, is one of these. He noticed a painless small lump in his right testicle, 2 months ago. He has only come to surgery because his wife insisted. He is quite embarrassed about the problem. You find that Simon's left testis is larger than the right but cannot identify a specific lump.

Questions: Simon
A. What is the differential diagnosis?
B. What is the likelihood of cancer?
C. What action do you take?
D. If it is cancer, will he be able to have a third child?

Answers: Simon
A. Although cancer is top of the list, you have to think of a hydrocoele (did you test for transillumination?), a torsion, orchitis (but usually painful), a spermatocoele or epididymal cyst (usually palpable separately from the testis) or the much rarer infections such as tuberculosis or syphilitic gummata.
B. The risk of cancer is quite high for an otherwise unexplained painless testicular swelling; over 50% in this age group will be cancer.
C. Urgent referral.** He is very likely to have an ultrasound taken at hospital but there is little to be gained in you organising this yourself.
D. This depends upon the treatment, which in itself depends upon the staging. Chemotherapy is likely to render him infertile but sperm collection and storage are possible before treatment.

** You probably think this was an easy decision, and it should have been. However, in the real case that this is derived from, no referral was made (and no notes were taken!). When Simon returned 7 months later, with a hard, heavy, lumpy testis, plus gynaecomastia, still no referral was made. It was a further year later, when the testis was painful, that the cancer was identified. It's easier on paper.

Case history 2
Irene

Still January and the country is in the grip of a flu-like bug. Irene (66) is no exception. Her illness began with a sore throat and myalgia and 'went on to her chest' 2 weeks ago, giving her a persistent cough. She blames this (as do you) on her five cigarettes a day. She produces yellow plugs of phlegm each morning but noticed a streak of blood in her sputum yesterday. Otherwise she's well, apart from being irritated that her bug has lasted so long. You can find nothing on examination.

Questions: Irene
A. What could be wrong with Irene? Can you put the possible diagnoses in a pecking order of likelihood?
B. Should you X-ray her?

Answers: Irene
A. This is a cancer book, so one of the answers is lung cancer. The chance is quite small – she smokes and has cough and haemoptysis but is otherwise well. In a non-smoker, the risk would be about 2.5%. It's twice that for Irene. A much likelier diagnosis is bronchitis, with a small blood vessel rupturing. Theoretically, it could be a pulmonary embolism or bronchiectasis or one of many other rare conditions. The fact she feels (and appears) well make these highly unlikely. The pecking order is tricky, as it will be chest infection first, no identifiable diagnosis second, lung cancer third and the others a distant fourth. What did you get in the sweepstake?
B. Would you agree to have a chest X-ray if your chance of lung cancer was 5%? Most people would. After all, a lung cancer won't go away and early diagnosis just might make a difference. All guidance suggests that an X-ray is indicated. In the real world, some patients and their GPs would be happy deferring the X-ray a week or so, to see if the haemoptysis recurs. Audits suggest that only half of patients with haemoptysis have a chest X-ray, so clearly GPs are deferring investigation in some instances (and largely correctly). This would be acceptable in a 40-year-old non-smoker but not so in Irene.

Case history 3
Tracy

Tracy is single, 28 and a receptionist at the local dental surgery. She doesn't come to the surgery much, other than for smears and for travel advice for her exotic foreign holidays. Her smear report arrives in your in-tray showing 'moderate dyskaryosis – referral recommended'.

Question: Tracy
A. What do you do?

Answer: Tracy
A. GPs have three main functions in the cervical screening programme. First, to organise both the taking of the smears and a watertight system of dealing with results. Second, to discuss their results with women, and third, to ensure referral when required. For Tracy, it is the latter two issues that are relevant.[+] You will want to discuss with her the natural history of abnormal cervical smears and the (uncomfortable) fact that she has quite advanced changes, for which treatment is recommended. The risk for Tracy of progression to cancer is probably higher than 1% a year. You will also want to make the referral for colposcopy and ensure it is prioritised.

[+] Of course, your practice system for receipt of smear results and action on abnormal results is watertight. Of course. . .

Case history 4
Ivor

Ivor is a manager in one of the local factories and is aged 53. He has executive screening as one of the 'perks' of his job. He has come to see you because the doctor at the screening medical found his PSA to be 4.7 ng/ml. The doctor has posted Ivor a printout of the results and recommended he see you for further investigation. He has no symptoms.

Questions: Ivor
A. What is the chance that Ivor has prostate cancer?
B. Should he have a transrectal ultrasound and biopsy? If so, will it hurt?
C. What happens if he does nothing?

Answers: Ivor
A. With a PSA over 4 ng/ml, the risk is somewhere between 24% and 38%, depending on which screening study you read. These risks are of course quite high but the real question is 'What is the risk of clinically significant cancer?', meaning one that actually poses a threat to life. No study has ever been able to put an accurate figure to that question but it is clearly less. Although you will make a referral, a rectal examination is appropriate, as you may be able to palpate an enlarged prostate or perhaps a nodule.
B. Most urologists would recommend these. The biopsy may be painful (though it may not) and patients may experience rectal bleeding afterwards. Several biopsies will be taken, as a cancer may be missed in a single core (or indeed in several cores).
C. If a cancer is found, one treatment option is 'watchful waiting', though this is less popular than it was. While the current evidence is not definitive, there may be small reductions in mortality when treated surgically. Ivor is young and the urologist is likely to recommend surgery or one of the newer treatments such as brachytherapy or high-frequency ultrasound. Even if the benefits of surgery prove to be real, the numbers needed to treat (NNTs) in the surgical trials were quite large, so doing nothing at the treatment stage is a reasonable option and, by extension, doing nothing at the diagnostic stage would be reasonable too. If such an option were chosen, regular PSAs would be wise.

Case history 5
Mabel

You hardly ever see Mabel and you have to check her thin records to see how old she is; 67, as it happens. She has consulted because she has had diarrhoea for a week, with 5–6 loose stools on her worst day but only two yesterday. There are no other symptoms and she appears well.

Questions: Mabel

A. On those facts alone, what do you think her risk of colorectal cancer is?

B. Is the fact that she hardly ever consults relevant?

You are sufficiently concerned to send a stool sample for microscopy and culture. Three days later the result returns. The microscopy shows red blood cells but there was no growth.

C. What is your plan?

Answers: Mabel

A. In a woman of 67, an isolated episode of diarrhoea is truly low risk. For the age group 40–70 the risk is about 0.5% when a patient reports diarrhoea to their GP, and in the over-70s it's around 1.3%.

B. This is a real pointer. Old-fashioned GP lore suggests you should be worried about two groups of people: the first is the low consulters, as they only come when something is *really* wrong with them and the second is the patient who returns with the same symptom, as you've clearly not cured them first time around. The first of these groups has been studied in general practice and thin-file patients are indeed at higher risk once they actually consult.[++]

C. Well done for sending a stool sample. Although no germs were grown, in practice you've done a faecal occult blood test and it's positive. The risk of cancer is now around 1 in 10 and you should refer urgently.

[++] Summerton N et al 2003 The general practitioner–patient consultation pattern as a tool for cancer diagnosis in general practice. British Journal of General Practice 53:50–52

Case history 6
Rafiq

Rafiq is 58, owns the best Indian restaurant in town and certainly enjoys his own cooking. He complains of weight loss over about 3 months but cannot put a figure on it. He's felt a little fatigued but is still working full time, which means he does more hours than his GP. You examine him very thoroughly but find nothing. He weighs 96 kg on the practice scales.

Questions: Rafiq

A. If you had to pick just one diagnosis, what would it be?
B. What investigations do you do?
C. If it is cancer, which sites are likely?

Answers: Rafiq

A. Sorry but type II diabetes must be top of the list. It's much more prevalent (and much more incident) than cancer. Both are more common with increasing age and although there is a link between obesity and some cancers, such as breast and colon, the link with diabetes is much stronger.

B. Maybe you made the diagnosis already by doing a urinalysis. If it were negative, then a full blood count, plus ESR or CRP, blood sugar, and perhaps liver and renal function tests, would be a reasonable start. If these are unhelpful and the weight loss continues, a PSA, faecal occult blood and a CXR would be the second-line tests. You may have to refer if no diagnosis has emerged from all these but even so, the risk of cancer in Rafiq will be quite small, perhaps only 1 in 10.

C. It could be almost any internal cancer, with colorectal, lung, prostate, upper GI and pancreas heading the list.

Case history 7
George

George is now 70. This is something of a success, as he consumed copious amounts of alcohol during his years as a travelling salesman, along with heavy smoking. He complains that food is sticking as he swallows and that he gets a brief pain behind his sternum with each swallow. He has no difficulty with liquids and has not lost weight. He has had his symptoms for about 3 weeks.

Questions: George
A. What possible diagnoses are in your mind?
B. What is your investigation plan?

Answers: George
A. George has localised his dysphagia to the lower oesophagus. In oesophageal disease the patient's location of the pain is usually quite accurate. Diseases of the lower oesophagus causing dysphagia for solids include oesophageal cancer, oesophageal stricture or spasm, and achalasia (though the latter is unlikely). A drug-induced ulcer can present this way. The oesophagus can be compressed externally, particularly by a lung tumour.
B. George should be referred for endoscopy urgently. There is little point in doing any primary care investigations.

Case history 8
Bethany

This delightful girl is 14 and her parents are justifiably proud of her. She's articulate, polite, popular and even keeps her bedroom tidy. Until last week, that is. It started with her saying she didn't want to go to school but being evasive in saying why. She just wanted to stay at home in bed. Her parents assumed there was an upset at school and their first response was to speak to Bethany's teacher, who could add little. She vomited this morning, so they have brought her as an extra at the end of morning surgery. On examination, she is a little withdrawn (she usually asks you questions, today she's passive) but you can't see much else. Fundoscopy is normal.

Questions: Bethany
A. This might be a brain tumour. What else could it be?
B. What do you do now?

Answers: Bethany
A. The differential diagnosis of a non-specifically ill child is wide and it's all rather vague – except the vomiting. The latter symptom makes non-organic ailments like school refusal much less likely. Infection, perhaps in the urinary tract, is possible but you would have expected some more focus to the symptoms. Gynaecological (or even obstetric!) problems are possible, as is anorexia. In short, the diagnosis is 'a sick kid'. Nothing wrong with that initial diagnosis, as long as you take steps to improve it.
B. You have little alternative but to refer her to a paediatrician, and today. Sure, the risk of a brain tumour is small but if you don't refer Bethany with these symptoms, you will never diagnose an early brain tumour in a child. In this case, it is better to be 'wrong' 99 times so that you are 'right' the one time. Posterior fossa tumours are very curable if diagnosed before irreversible brain damage has occurred.

Case history 9
Edgar

Edgar is 82 and copes well with his type II diabetes, mild hypertension and joint aches. He is a reliable attender for his check-ups. Your practice arrangements for diabetic review are that he sees the practice nurse first for blood and urine testing and you review him with the results. This time, however, urinalysis has shown 2+ of blood as well as + proteinuria.

Questions: Edgar

A. What do you do about the haematuria in primary care?

B. The urine contains several red blood cells and culture is negative. How do you investigate now?

Answers: Edgar

A. The initial thing is to confirm the haematuria, by sending a sample for microscopy and culture. The test sticks for haematuria are very sensitive and it may be that that no blood is seen on confirmatory testing. There is little point in doing cytology, as the test sensitivity is too low for a negative test to provide adequate reassurance. Even if the result were positive, Edgar will still need a cystoscopy, so you've not saved him any trouble.

B. Edgar should be referred for investigation. The urologist will probably request an ultrasound and perform a cystoscopy. The risk of cancer with haematuria at Edgar's age is quite high, probably in the order of 25%. Most of these will be bladder tumours, and so very treatable, though prostate and kidney cancer are also possible.

Case history 10
Ian

Ian is a 35-year-old forester, with muscular arms like the tree trunks he saws down. He has noticed a dark lesion on his upper chest, which at first he blamed on his protective clothing rubbing. The lesion is shown in Figure 18.1.

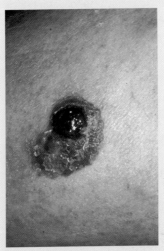

Figure 18.1   The skin lesion on Ian's chest (photo courtesy of Ian Daniels).

Questions: Ian
A. Does this look like a nodular malignant melanoma? Will you excise it or refer?
B. Histology confirms this as a melanoma. Ian asks if he can continue in his job, as he is outside all day. What do you think?

Answers: Ian
A. This is a classic nodular malignant melanoma. It should not be excised in primary care. Indeed, if there is any suspicion of cancer, referral is wiser than excision in the surgery.
B. There is no doubt he is at increased risk.[*+] In patients with no predisposing factors, the risk of developing a second (or subsequent)

[*+] Goggins W, Tsao H 2003 A population-based analysis of risk factors for a second primary cutaneous melanoma among melanoma survivors. Cancer 97:639–643 melanoma is 1% after 1 year, 3% at 10 years and 5% at 20 years. The risk is higher in older patients, men and those with the first melanoma on the trunk, face or neck. Whether this translates into recommending that Ian stops outdoor work (just how practical is this in a 35-year-old forester?) is a moot point even for the most self-confident GP. Some of the increased risk is probably genetic in origin, though that doesn't mean he can ignore the additional risk from excess sun exposure. Clearly, he needs to be strict in protecting himself from the sun with sunscreens and wearing a long-sleeved shirt at all times.

Case history 11
Eileen

Eileen has unconventional medical views, preferring to consult alternative practitioners on the few occasions she is ill. She has reached the age of 55 in rude health, which has confirmed her in her view of the superiority of complementary therapies. She doesn't attend for smears or mammography. She had a benign breast lump excised some years ago. She attends, asking for examination of her breast, as she thinks another lump has developed. Sure enough, you feel a spherical lump about 1.5 cm across, which is fluctuant and semi-mobile. You advise Eileen that she needs to see a specialist but she flatly refuses, saying she will seek treatment of her problem with one of her alternative practitioners.

Questions: Eileen
A. What is her risk of cancer with this breast lump?
B. Have you any primary care options in the face of her refusal to accept conventional referral?

Nine months later Eileen reattends and her breast problem has advanced, to the state shown in Figure 18.2. This is clearly malignant, though there are no palpable secondaries. You tell her it is cancer and she says emphatically she will not have surgery.

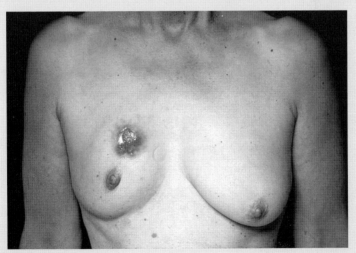

Figure 18.2   Breast cancer (photo courtesy of Ian Daniels).

C. What options do you have now?

Answers: Eileen

A. It is difficult to be accurate about the actual risk. Various figures have been stated, like 'nine out of ten breast lumps are benign', but (perhaps not surprisingly) no primary care study has actually calculated a figure. One thing is clear, however. Once a lump is present, the risk factors, such as a family history or a previous benign lump, do not matter. The lump is present and it is the lump that carries the risk.

B. Clearly, you would strongly advise seeing a surgeon. If her reluctance is simply to do with fear of a biopsy (it's not, of course) then there are some alternatives. One study of women with a lump followed those who had negative mammograms and ultrasounds (both tests showing normal breast tissue at the site of the lump) but who did not have a biopsy; no cancers developed in the next 2 years. An alternative would be to aspirate this possible cyst. Although cysts and cancers can co-exist, the risk is much smaller once fluid has been found. Even so, you would be wise to discuss her with secondary care.

C. You are out of your depth here. It is not reasonable to expect a GP to know all therapeutic options. You will need to get specialist help. The specialist may be able to suggest radiotherapy, chemotherapy or hormonal manipulation. The key thing is that the woman is perfectly entitled to make her own decisions, however wacky you think they are.

In the real case on which this was based, the 'blame' lay with the GP. Although the patient refused an aspiration at the initial consultation, no referral was made and none was made on two subsequent occasions when a lump was still palpable. The patient is dead.

Case history 12
Susan

Susan is 78 and complaining of dysuria, along with vaginal and vulval pain. She is a moderately well-controlled diabetic. You examine her external genitalia and what you see is shown in Figure 18.3.

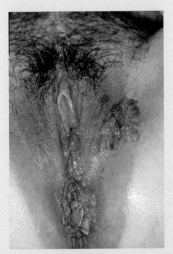

Figure 18.3   Vulval ulceration (photo courtesy of Ian Daniels).

Questions: Susan
A. Could this be a florid fungal infection?
B. What is your management plan?

Answers: Susan
A. There may be some superadded candida infection but this cannot possibly explain the ulceration. This is a vulval cancer.
B. She should be referred urgently to a gynaecological oncologist.

Case history 13
Colin

Colin is a 66-year-old retired plumber. His cousin has been diagnosed as suffering from a rare, inherited haematological condition and he wants to know if he has it too. As part of the work-up, a full blood count and serum ferritin are taken. The tests show that Colin hasn't inherited the condition but also reveal borderline anaemia, with a significantly low serum ferritin.

Question: Colin
A. What do you do to investigate the abnormal blood results?

Answer: Colin
A. Colin has mild anaemia and a low iron. Although there are other causes of iron deficiency anaemia (including diet, angiodysplasia and peptic ulceration), it is mandatory to investigate the gastrointestinal tract. Arguments rage about whether it is better to do top first (gastroscopy) or bottom first (colonoscopy). In truth, both will be needed most of the time, as only about 10% will be due to a colorectal cancer and less will be due to a gastric lesion. The ugly fact is that only about half of patients presenting to primary care with iron deficiency anaemia are referred for gastrointestinal investigation.

Case history 14
Vera

Vera is a very popular patient with the practice, not just because she brings chocolate bars to the surgery every time she consults. She never married, staying at home to look after her elderly mother, who died a few years ago. Vera is 73 and a lifelong non-smoker. She is hoarse, though only partially so and you can make out her story. The problem began 5 weeks ago with a cold, which she shrugged off but she has never really regained the strength of her voice. There is nothing to find on examining her throat or her chest.

Question: Vera
A. What is your plan for 5 weeks of partial hoarseness?

Answer: Vera
A. The risk of cancer with hoarseness is probably below 1%. However, Vera has been hoarse for 5 weeks, even though she has still some voice. The chance of this being laryngitis is diminishing. Indeed, referral guidance uses 3 weeks as the threshold for referral, though most GPs would wait a little longer if the symptoms were improving.

    The initial investigation is a CXR, as lung cancer is more common than laryngeal cancer. However, in Vera's case lung cancer is quite unlikely as there are no other symptoms or signs. There is a good case for skipping the CXR and making an urgent ENT referral now.

Index